P9-DWU-405

Stress
for
Success

By the same author

Suddenly Silence
Rimu, Hamilton, New Zealand, 1998

Stress
for
Success

How to Cope with Stress and Enjoy Life

Ilene Birkwood

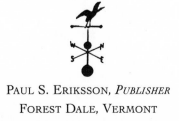

PAUL S. ERIKSSON, *PUBLISHER*
FOREST DALE, VERMONT

© 1999 by Ilene Birkwood

All rights reserved. No part of this work may be reproduced
in any form without permission in writing from
Paul S. Eriksson, *Publisher*, Post Office Box 125,
Forest Dale, Vermont 05745.

Manufactured in the United States of America

5 4 3 2 1

Library of Congress Cataloging-in-Publication Data
Birkwood, Ilene
Stress for sucess: how to cope with stress
and enjoy life / by Ilene Birkwood.
p. cm.
Originally published: Mangonui, N.Z.: Shoreline Press, 1996.
ISBN 0-8397-7930-5 (pbk.)
1. Stress management. 2. Stress (Phychology) I. Title.
RA785.B57   1999
155.9'042–DC21   99-24440
CIP

Designed by Eugenie S. Delaney

Acknowledgments

❧❧❧

The author wishes to express her thanks to Lyn Anderson, Des Gotobed, and Sally and Peter Lawton for their help and encouragement during the preparation of this book. In addition, I would like to give special thanks to Jill Smith of the Kaeo Medical Centre and Debbie Francis of Relationship Services for their assistance and sound advice, and in particular, I would like to thank my friend LeJeune Whitney for her invaluable assistance.

The ideas and techniques presented in this book are things the author has found to be beneficial in reducing the effects of stress. Neither the author, editor nor publisher are members of the medical profession, nor are they practitioners of alternative medicine. While every effort has been made to present accurate and helpful information, the author, editor, and publisher disclaim liability to any person for the consequences of anything done by them in reliance upon any part of the contents of this publication.

Contents

❧❦

Introduction

This book provides a practical guide to dealing with stress. By helping you understand stress, it will show you how to combat its effects. A series of simple procedures, that take no more than a few minutes each day, can have a major impact on the quality of your lifestyle. It is possible to lessen the effects of chronic stress—insomnia, headaches, clenched jaws, constant fatigue—immediately and eventually get you to the point where you can enjoy life to the full. Stress will have been reduced to a pleasant stimulant rather than a monster overshadowing your life.

Since lack of time is probably one of the factors that contributes to your stress level, the techniques selected are ones that fit into the busiest schedule. They are simple to learn, and you will feel up to coping with them even after the most brain-numbing day.

Four fundamentals form the basis of stress control:

Counteracting the Effects of a Stressful Situation

Your body initiates a "fight or flight" reaction when you are faced with a stressful situation. Stress reaction is a primitive response to a threatening or dangerous situation and has been important in ensuring the survival of the human species. Survival has depended on man's ability to fight or outrun his attacker. The threat of attack causes changes in body chemistry, increasing alertness, muscular strength and speed to prepare for a physical showdown, or hasty retreat. This fight or flight response causes an increase in blood pressure, a faster heart rate, higher levels of blood fats and increases the clotting ability of the blood to plug up wounds. After the emergency, the body returns to its normal relaxed state.

Unfortunately, when we are subjected to long-term psychological stress, our body still initiates the stone-age fight or flight response. We are ready for physical action but cannot beat our manager over the head or run out of a meeting. Consequently, we bottle up our emotions and keep our cool. The resulting anxiety is felt as a state of chronic readiness; we cannot relax. Without physical release, our body stays on red alert for extended periods, leaving us tense and exhausted.

However, you can counteract this by initiating the relaxation response. The fight or flight reaction programs your body for action. The relaxation response deprograms it, dissipating the effects of stress before it can harm you.

The relaxation response is based on the principle of muscular relaxation. When you are anxious or disturbed your muscles tense. Conversely, when your muscles relax, the mind relaxes, and the tension caused by stress fades away. In Chapter 3 this is explained in more detail, and methods are described which initiate the relaxation response. None of the methods explained take more than a few minutes to learn.

Stressful Situations Do Not Cause Problems

Stressful situations do not cause problems. It is your reaction to the situation that causes them. Stress occurs within your mind. By learning to view stress differently you can nullify its effect.

Stress will always be with us whatever our age and occupation. Software experts, housepersons, airline pilots, mail carriers, managers, retired people and physicists all suffer from stress. Fortunately, stressful situations (which are generally outside our control) do not cause the problem; it is our reaction to the situation (which is under our control) that causes emotional and physical problems. Once we learn to control our reactions, we have dramatically dampened the effects of stress.

Your perception of a situation affects the stress level experienced by your body. If your mind screams "Red Alert! Red Alert!" whenever you are confronted with a stressful situation, your body works overtime pumping adrenalin. However, if your mind says, "Oh, hell, here comes more stress. No problem. I know how to cope," your body's reaction is mild. It is not so much your actual ability to cope with a situation as much as your *perception* of your ability to cope.

To Combat the Effects of Stress You Need to Tune Up Your Body

Our body has remarkable healing powers. Just as chronic mental stress produces unpleasant side effects such as headaches, tense muscles and an upset stomach, a relaxed mind and body can produce the opposite, and reverse these effects.

Subjecting your body to constant stress without treating it right is a bit like buying a BMW and constantly driving full bore without ever having it tuned. To say nothing of frequently filling it with the wrong fuel. Would you really expect it to continue to operate at optimum performance? Since you don't treat your car that badly, don't you think it's time to start giving your body equal time?

If you look after your body and treat it right, it will be a powerful weapon in the fight against stress. Paying attention to your diet (feeding it the correct fuel) and giving it fresh air and exercise (tuning it) will pay tremendous dividends in increased energy, sound sleep and a capacity for enjoyment. The exercises suggested are all well within the capabilities of the most avid couch potato, and the diet suggestions center on good nutrition rather than rigid slimming.

You are the Key Factor

One other issue needs to be addressed, and that is your mindset. *You have to take responsibility for your own body and your own life.* Doctors can prescribe pills that deal with the symptoms of stress, but only you can treat the cause. And until you address the causes, both internal and external, stresses will continue to take their toll. Pills bring only temporary relief and will need to be taken in increasing doses if chronic stress continues.

If stress is already a constant factor in your life, then you also probably suffer from fatigue. Stress is one of the primary causes of chronic tiredness. However, if you start using the techniques described, you can begin to combat tiredness and find a new fund of energy. For example, taking a twenty-minute walk at lunchtime will start to tap into your body's latent energy. With increased energy you will be able to gradually increase the number of stress-preventing techniques described, and you are then on an upward spiral to a healthy, well-balanced life. One where you have time to tackle your work with enthusiasm, spend more time on relationships and enjoy your leisure.

ONE

Stress in Perspective

"If you don't know what to do next, walk fast and look worried."

By practicing a few simple procedures, you can learn to control stress. Stress causes problems—physically, emotionally and mentally. What is more it prevents you from enjoying life to the full. Even when you are in a job you love, and in a happy relationship, the sheer number of day-to-day problems, and the accompanying time pressures, create a stress level that leaves you exhausted at the end of the day. Sometimes even whipping up the energy to have a good time on the weekend takes strength of character. Compound this with a job you dislike, and relationship problems, and stress becomes overwhelming.

However, it doesn't have to be that way. By investing about forty minutes a day, you can start enjoying a balanced, relaxed lifestyle even in a stress-filled environment.

We all know people who sail through life apparently unaffected by stress. They always seem to be in control and regard each new stressful situation as a challenge to be overcome rather than a crippling blow. These lucky few, as a result of genes, upbringing and environment, have a natural immunity to stress. Fortunately, the skills that come naturally to the lucky few are skills that can be acquired with practice. By understanding the nature of stress, and by learning to control your reaction to it, you can learn to cope with even chronic, unremitting stress.

Stress is a complex entity made up of a variety of components, and the stress you feel is a direct result of this makeup. You are subjected to external stresses such as constant interruptions, red traffic lights or a crying baby, and internal stresses such as anger, fear or resentment. Your reaction to these stresses is affected by your state of mind at the time, your physical state and such mundane items as how well you slept the night before.

Once you understand stress and how it affects you, you can learn how to deal with it. And as you begin to practice your new-found skills, you will start to enjoy life.

Stress — the Myth

Somewhere along the line stress has picked up a bad name. Most of the ailments of modern mankind are blamed on stress. The medical profession blames it for everything from ingrowing toenails to leukemia. As your unanswered E-mail grows exponentially, the phone rings incessantly, and you know you'll never make it home in time for your child's birthday party, you tend to agree with them. It feels as if stress is this huge monster poised to devour you.

Once you learn how to deal with stress—and it isn't that difficult—you'll get it into perspective. It's not a monster threatening to ruin your life. It's a pleasant stimulant that adds zest to life and keeps you functioning at peak performance.

You are Unique

A lot has been written about stress. Just run to your local bookstore and look at the shelves groaning with the collective wisdom of doctors, retired executives, psychologists and management consultants. You can gain a lot of help from reading them. However, most of them tend to overlook one basic essential. No two people are alike. We all react to stress differently. So universal recipes for dealing with stress don't always work.

You are a unique person with your own personality, likes and dislikes. This book will provide information on how you can deal with stress. From the various techniques suggested you can find your own unique formula. By selecting techniques that appeal to you, and which can be incorporated into your lifestyle, you can establish a routine that you will enjoy. And in addition you will feel better, sleep better and stay healthier.

I would encourage you to practice those methods that appeal to you, because those are the ones that you will continue to use regularly.

Sit back and enjoy the book and try those things that appeal to you. And if you feel just too tired to bother to select for yourself, you'll find a step-by-step approach set out for you in Chapter 11.

What This Book Will Provide

This book provides an overview of the best of the anti-stress solutions offered today, including aromatherapy, reflexology, meditation and massage. It addresses diet (healthy eating vs. calorie counting), exercise and the importance of restful sleep and relaxation. It will talk about the benefits of walking in the forest or beside the ocean, listening to classical music and soaking in a warm, aromatic tub after a hard day's work.

From the major anti-stress solutions, I have selected several quick and easy things you can do immediately to improve your situation. If you wish to delve further into any area that seems tailor-made for you, information is provided so that you can continue. This might be where to purchase the essential oils needed for aromatherapy, how to contact a Reflexologist, or how to find more information on yoga or meditation.

No one thing will necessarily provide the solution, but a combination of techniques borrowed from several disciplines can make a major difference. Decide which of the techniques appeal to you.

I have also referred to books that provide more information on each subject. However, there is nothing sacred about my recommendations. Don't elevate your stress level by a frantic search. Simply go to a large bookstore and ask for recommendations, or let them point you in the direction of the right shelf. Then browse for a while. There are lots of books on each subject. Find one that has an approach you like.

I am very aware of how busy you are. In all probability, the fact that you have so little time to yourself is one of the causes of your stress. So, from the innumerable stress remedies available, this book will present the ones that provide the maximum effect for the minimum amount of time and effort. Several of them can be started right away.

None of them take more than twenty minutes or so. Others take a little longer and require some preparation. However, with the information provided you can decide which of them to pursue. To keep functioning at peak performance you have to feel good about yourself. By taking a small amount of time each day to improve your health and sense of well-being, you'll be surprised how much time you suddenly have to spare.

And, more importantly, you are going to find the quality of your life has improved dramatically. You will still be working just as hard, and in all probability you will still be subjected to all manner of stress, but with an increased capacity to cope, and a more balanced lifestyle, stress will no longer be a major factor in your life.

All the techniques described will help you relax and cope with stress. However, if you are suffering from severe stress, or any other ailment, I would urge you to consult a doctor. The techniques described can be a powerful complement in medical treatment, but they are not a substitute.

TWO

What Is Stress?

The word stress is derived from the Latin word *stringere* which means "to draw tight." So uptight accurately describes the response to stress. Stress reaction is a primitive response to a threatening or dangerous situation, causing changes in our body chemistry. After the emergency our body should return to its normal, relaxed state. Unfortunately, when we are subjected to long-term psychological stress this does not happen. Instead we are in a state of chronic readiness; we cannot relax. Without physical release, our body stays on red alert for extended periods, leaving us feeling tense and exhausted.

The Answer to Stress

The answer to stress is to bring your body back into balance as quickly as possible after it has been subjected to a stressful situation. By initiating the relaxation response you can immediately dampen the effects of psychological stress. For example, the relaxation response can be initiated by simple and immediate remedies such as deep breathing or taking a short walk. However, how you initiate the relaxation response to counteract the adverse effects of the fight or flight syndrome will be the subject of several of the following chapters.

Reaction to Stress

Treatment of the symptoms of stress only bring short-term relief. For permanent relief, you have to address the causes. Since many of these causes are outside your control, you need to look at them differently—and this is where your reaction to stress is important. You may not be able to control the cause of your stress, but you can gradually learn to control your reaction to it.

There's an old story about a man who was moving West with his family. As his covered wagon entered a small town, he saw an old man leaning on a gate.

The traveler asked, "What are the people like who live in this town?"

The old man looked up and asked, "What were people like in your home town?"

The traveler replied, "They were great. Very kind-hearted and hospitable. We hated to leave, but there just wasn't any work."

The old man nodded, and said, "Yes, you'll find the people in this town much the same."

The man thanked him and continued into town.

A few days later another traveler came into town and seeing the old man, still leaning on the gate, asked, "What type of people live here?"

The old man replied as before, "What were people like in your home town?"

The traveler answered, "Oh, they were a miserable lot. Bad tempered and always finding fault. I was glad to be out of there."

The old man nodded and said, "Yes, you'll find them just the same here. I should look elsewhere if I were you."

The story illustrates how our perception of life dictates how we experience events in life. It is no different with stress. It is not so much your actual ability to cope with a situation as much as your perception of your ability to cope.

We cannot alter the stresses of life; most of them will be with us for a long time. However, we can train ourselves to deal with them so that as each stressful situation arises you perceive it in a totally different way. Relaxation techniques, meditation, diet and exercise all help control and decrease the stress response. And, as you grow increasingly confident in your ability to control the stress response, you perceive stress as a diminishing threat, and your body responds by steadily decreasing the stress response.

You are the Key

The first step in getting stress under control is for you to make up your mind that you are going to learn how to deal with stress and that it is going to be a constantly diminishing problem from here on in.

Your attitude will make a difference. From the minute

you feel positive about yourself, and start sending your body the right signals, it will respond. The body is a bit like a computer—it only delivers what it is programmed to do. If you keep telling yourself, "I can't stand the strain; if the phone rings again or the baby cries, I'll scream," your brain feeds all these negative thoughts to your poor body which responds the way you're expecting it to, with knots in the stomach, headaches and insomnia.

Similarly, we all have ingrained attitudes and behavioral responses to everyday situations. If we fume and slap the dashboard each time a traffic light turns red, this is something we have been doing for years in all probability. Our behavioral responses can be adjusted too. Somewhere along the way we learned our behavior patterns. Now that we are smart adults, we can just as easily teach ourselves new patterns. So start thinking right. Send positive signals to your body. Eventually it will become second nature.

> If as you are reading this you are absolutely dog-tired, and all you really want to do is crawl under the covers and sleep for a week, then flip to Chapter 4. Pick up some ideas on how to get a good, refreshing night's sleep. Then read the rest of this book at your leisure.

Stress Checklist

Make a list of the things that create the most stress in your life. Check the ones below that apply, then write out your own list.

- Non-stop phone calls
- Red traffic lights when you're in a hurry
- A new job
- Constant interruptions
- Sales phone calls
- Meetings
- Overflowing in-basket
- People who are late for appointments
- Your partner's snoring
- Not being able to eat your favorite food because you're dieting
- Copy machine jamming
- System going down
- Boss pressuring you
- Out of town relatives staying with you
- Not having enough money to meet expenses
- Car not starting
- Car out of gas
- Not getting enough sleep

_____

_____

_____

_____

_____

_____

_____

_____

_____

_____

_____ continue list.

After you've completed the list, take ten minutes to review it. If you really look at it, you'll find several things you could eliminate. Maybe getting household help or reorganizing your work day would do it, or planning to leave a couple of minutes earlier for appointments to avoid frustration when you're held up en route. Dozens of books have been written on time management, so we won't get into most of those issues. But reducing the length of the list will automatically reduce your stress level.

Things You Enjoy Doing

Now make a list of the things you like to do most. Here are a few suggestions; check those that apply, then continue with your own list:

- Walking in the park
- Going to the movies
- Reading a mystery novel
- Spending time with the kids
- Playing golf
- Playing tennis
- Jogging
- Listening to opera music
- Going to the theatre
- Going out to dinner
- Doing crosswords
- Surfing the Internet
- Looking at the stars
- Cooking gourmet meals
- Gardening
- Playing with the dog

_____

_____

_____

_____

_____

_____

_____

_____

_____

_____

_____ continue list.

Now review the list. Are you taking time to do any of these things? Why not? You need to have balance in your life. Think about how you could make the time to do something you enjoy each day. How do you know if any of the things you enjoy are helping with stress? It's very simple. You'll feel good. You'll forget work. Your body will feel calm and relaxed.

THREE

Techniques for Dealing with Stress

❦

Before we get down to talking about the techniques you can use to strengthen your resistance to stress, let's talk about realistic expectations. Do you honestly believe that every plane is going to leave on time? That all your friends and business associates are going to turn up on time for an appointment? That every traffic light is going to be green?

Of course you don't. However, each and every time one of these things happen, you grow agitated, and make yourself angrier and angrier the longer the situation continues. The plane hasn't even arrived at the departure gate, but already you are pacing up and down looking at your watch.

By the time the delayed flight touches down, the cleaners have done their thing and the plane has been okayed for takeoff, you have induced in yourself a steady, burning anger. Imagine what that is doing to your stress level.

So get realistic with your expectations. When the plane is delayed, settle down to do some work, or have a cup of coffee. When the traffic light is red, turn on some soothing music, or practice your breathing exercises. When your friend is late yet again, smile and say, "I love him in spite of his tardy nature," or get a new friend.

Mind and Body

Although science likes to compartmentalize the mind and body, there is a very real connection between the two. How you think and feel determines how your body deals with stress. Anxiety and muscle tension go hand in hand. When you are alert and on guard, the muscles tense for action. The body language of an angry person illustrates this clearly. Conversely, when your muscles relax, they induce a feeling of calm.

To counteract the effects of stress, you need to relax. Some people find this easy. Others don't. Fortunately, you can learn how to relax if it doesn't come easily. When you learn how to recognize muscle tension, you can learn how to relax tense muscles and enjoy the accompanying calmness of mind this induces. Learning to relax is powerfully therapeutic.

You will find your powers of concentration improve, small irritations become less important, and you will stop feeling tired all the time. When you do become tired, it will be a healthy tiredness which can be overcome with refreshing, undisturbed sleep.

Relaxation can be achieved by a variety of techniques—some physical, some mental. Since physical techniques will have a more immediate appeal if you are in a very hyper, stressed-out state, unable to relax for more than few minutes at a time, I will start there.

The physical approach allows you to be "doing something" which in your present state is essential for every waking moment. By exercising and deep breathing you will be able to achieve a pleasant level of relaxation which will improve your ability to sleep and leave you refreshed and calm. You can then progress to meditation if you wish. With meditation you can achieve the same level of relaxation and also build an inner reservoir of calm.

Whether the approach is physical, mental or sensual, all the techniques outlined will put you on the road to relaxation. And with relaxation comes a fuller enjoyment of life and an ability to shrug off the stresses of the day.

Initiating the Relaxation Response

Two of the simplest ways of initiating the relaxation response are by exercising and by controlled breathing.

Exercise

Exercise is of major importance in reducing stress. The type of exercise you choose should be something you enjoy doing. Because if you enjoy it you will keep it up, and it is important that you do it regularly. You should aim to exercise at least three times a week but preferably every day.

Exercise is good at any time. Most people exercise first

thing in the morning, after work or before dinner. The advantage of early morning is that you have more control over your schedule and it becomes part of your daily routine. It also makes you start the day feeling good, physically relaxed and ready for anything. Then, of course, there's that slightly smug feeling you enjoy as you finish your run just as the rest of the world is stumbling out of bed.

Activity is essential to life. If we stay in one position for a long time, we experience pain and fatigue. Muscles benefit from movement and need the good circulation it promotes. Movement directly induces relaxation because muscle groups work in pairs, one relaxing as the opposing group tenses. If muscles are held tight and tense in one position for any length of time, the circulation is impeded, and the fatigue by-product, lactic acid, accumulates, leading to numerous aches and pains. These are felt particularly in the muscles of the neck and shoulders.

Sustained muscle tension frequently goes unnoticed; tight shoulders, clenched jaws, clenched fists, gripped thumb and furrowed brow all become habitual to the point that you are unaware of them. Exercise will release the tension from your muscles.

The exercise should be one that uses the main muscle groups, especially the legs, in a rhythmic fashion. Walking, swimming, jogging and cycling are all excellent. Find something that will fit into your daily routine—a twenty-minute walk or a swim at lunchtime will do you more good than sitting with your feet up drinking a cup of coffee. Remember, exercise should refresh you and help you enjoy the rest of the day. It should not be a mind-numbing, exhausting experience.

Highly competitive sports, while exhilarating, are not the optimum in reducing stress. Select exercise that is enjoyable but does not increase your tension level. For example, if you're an uptight golfer (and I've known golfers who take tranquilizers before they play), golf, in spite of all the advantages of providing exercise in the open air, will probably not help you too much. If, on the other hand, you thoroughly enjoy golf and have a relaxed attitude, go for it.

Exercise makes you feel good, stimulates your circulation and refreshes your mind. It also releases the tension that builds up in your muscles in a stress-filled day. Stress causes your muscles to tense up. Exercise releases that tension, and the muscles send signals to the brain to relax. Exercise, particularly in the fresh air, will also improve the quality of your sleep, but don't exercise just before bedtime. It is too stimulating.

Walking on the beach is a great form of exercise. Sea air makes you feel wonderful, and the ocean has a calming effect. Even on a still day the sea is restless, always on the move, so watch it and relax—the sea has taken over.

Setting the Stage for Relaxation

Learning to deal with stress is all about learning how to relax. To learn to relax you need to set the stage. Once you have learned the procedures and have them down pat you will be able to practice them anywhere, in flight departure lounges, in the office, in a taxi or while waiting at traffic lights. In the meantime, it pays to sit or lie comfortably, to wear comfortable clothing and to find a quiet, private environment. You should be behind a closed door and away from the sound of the phone and doorbell.

Regularity and repetition are also important. You need to start practicing the techniques on a regular basis. But don't practice them within two hours of a full meal. Relaxation techniques will probably cause you to drop off to sleep.

Thought Control

The relaxation response can be initiated by gaining control of your thoughts and blocking out the disturbing thoughts that cause problems. Learning thought control is difficult, and it is an area where practice is most needed. The most effective method is to direct attention away from your normal thought pattern. We can't totally concentrate on two things at the same time, and if we learn to concentrate on something we can block other thoughts. One of the ways of doing this is by concentrating on your breathing. One of the most commonly known examples of breathing techniques is that used during childbirth where the mother is taught to concentrate on her breathing to drive the pain to a position of secondary importance. Don't worry, the type of breathing I am going to recommend is the type you can do in public without drawing attention to yourself—not the intense type used so often in hospital dramas.

Breathing

Although we all know breathing is related to our emotions—breath coming faster in alarming situations for example—the converse, that regular, slow, deep breaths may banish tension, is not generally recognized. Taking a number of slow, deep breaths and exhaling gently will calm you down and release tension.

Breathing is one of the vital functions over which we can exercise conscious control, and because of its close connection with our emotions we are able to quiet down our emotional response by controlling our breathing. Breathing exercises teach you to breathe fully so that you can quietly and unobtrusively fill your lungs and exhale slowly in stressful situations. This will overcome the tendency to shallow tension-filled breathing which heightens your anxiety level.

A very simple exercise is to breathe in slowly as you count up to seven, and then exhale slowly counting from one to 15. As you breathe in, push out your abdomen and feel the oxygen expanding your chest, then as you slowly exhale, feel all the tension drain out of you. Repeat this five or more times.

Initially, you may find it hard to exhale more slowly than you inhale. That's okay. Simply aim to count one more on exhaling; inhale on the count of seven, exhale on count of eight. You will find with practice that you will be able to gradually extend it. Ask a singer or an actor to demonstrate, and they'll inhale on the count of seven and exhale on the count of 60!

This very calming exercise has a huge advantage over all others. You can do it anywhere without anyone knowing what you are doing. When you're just going in for an interview, or are about to make a presentation, take a few minutes and several deep breaths. The chances of becoming tense and anxious will be reduced significantly, and you'll feel cool and calm on center stage.

KEEPING IN BALANCE

STRESS

Relaxation Response

Body prepared

Body's natural release of stress encouraged by:

Exercise

Diet

Controlled Breathing

Aromatherapy

Meditation

Reflexology

Laughter

Music

FIGHT OR FLIGHT

Tense muscles, Insomnia, Headaches, Upset stomach, Irritability, High blood pressure

---

The key to using this method successfully is a slow, relatively short inhalation phase, followed by a slow, controlled, longer exhalation phase. Try to breathe in for two to three seconds, pause briefly, then exhale for three to four seconds. Concentrate on the breathing out phase, gently expelling all the air from your lungs. Don't blow the air out in one short puff and then hold your breath. It is the slow exhalation process that induces calm. Practice this for a few days, then try gradually extending the time to breathe out.

Breathing — Part II

Another breathing exercise that will help you relax follows. I wouldn't recommend doing this one in public.

- Lie down, or sit in a comfortable chair.
- Clench your feet as tightly as you can and breathe in.
- Clench your feet even tighter.
- Then slowly unclench your feet, exhaling gently.
- Next, clench your calf muscles and breathe in.
- Clench your calf muscles even tighter.
- Unclench your muscles and exhale gently.
- Work your way through all the major muscle groups in your body: legs, stomach, hands, arms, not forgetting your face muscles.
- Really screw up those eyes.
- If your calf muscles start to go into cramp, relax them immediately and move on to another muscle group.

After you have done this exercise two or three times, you will find all your muscles have relaxed, and with muscular release comes the lessening of tension. Just as your mind signals your body to tense up in stressful situations, your muscles signal your mind to relax.

The object of this exercise, by the way, is not to create wrinkles in your face but to make you aware of how tense your muscles are. Chronic stress produces muscles tight with tension and, because you live with it every day, you no longer realize how tense your muscles are. If you practice this exercise regularly, you will begin to recognize the difference between tense and relaxed muscles. And armed with that knowledge, you can release the tension before it has time to build up and cause you problems.

Before Bed

To relax your muscles and relieve your anxieties before going to bed, try the following (you will find falling asleep a great deal easier once you are relaxed):

1. Stretch the rib cage and spine using overhead arm stretches, rock from side to side, then clasp hands behind your back and lift to fully expand the chest area.

2. Next, inhale on the count of five. Concentrate on filling the lower lungs. Place your hands on your abdomen, feeling it expand.

3. Exhale slowly on the count of seven, relaxing totally and emptying your lungs. Concentrate on your abdomen, feeling it contract.

Repeat the exercise several times, breathing very slowly and concentrating on each breath.

To improve respiration, you can also use a vaporizer with a few drops of lemon essential oil, tea tree and thyme, or alternatively cedarwood essential oil, eucalyptus and tea tree. (Essential oils are discussed in Chapter 5.)

Yoga and Breathing

Hatha Yoga, the form most frequently practiced in the West, concentrates on three main aspects—posture, breathing and meditation. Exercises are designed to improve posture and breathing on the principle that these lead to improved physical health as well as greater confidence and serenity because stress and tension are removed.

Three simple Hatha Yoga exercises you can do at home are: breathing, neck roll and shoulder roll.

I. BREATHING

Kneel down. Put your thumbs and index fingers together. Completely empty the lungs. Now gently breathe in on the count of seven and out on the count of seven. Repeat for about three times morning and evening. It is important to be comfortable while you are kneeling and not to put any undue stress on your knees or feet. If it is uncomfortable kneeling on the floor, then kneel on a pillow.

2. NECK ROLL

Kneeling in the same position, let your head fall towards your chest, then rotate the head slowly and smoothly clockwise three times and anti-clockwise three times. Move only your neck; keep your shoulders still. This relieves tension in the neck area.

Try this one very carefully and gently initially. If it feels comfortable the first time through, then continue. However, if you feel even the slightest discomfort, discontinue and try the following.

Move your head to look over your left shoulder, hold it for a second, then move your head to look over your right shoulder. Repeat twice. Do not look any farther than is comfortable.

Now tuck your chin down towards your breastbone. Raise your head slowly and look above your head. Repeat twice.

The object of the exercise is to loosen up your neck muscles, which are a seat of tension.

3. SHOULDER ROLL

Kneel down, with your arms at your sides. With your arms hanging down, slowly rotate each arm clockwise three times and anti-clockwise three times. Repeat.

For more information on Yoga, refer to the following books:

Yoga The Iyengar Way by Silva, Mira and Shyam Mehta. Published by Simon & Schuster.

Yoga by Kay Martin and Judy Charlesworth. Published by Penguin Books.

Yoga by Chris Stevens. Published by A. & C. Black.

The Book of Yoga by Lucy Liddell. Published by Ebury Press.

Yoga is extremely relaxing and with its emphasis on controlled breathing, balance and inner calm, it can make a major impact on your stress level. If you are interested in practicing yoga, I would strongly recommend taking a course from a qualified instructor.

FOUR

Sleep

Probably one of the worst manifestations of stress is not being able to get to sleep at night, or waking up in the middle of the night with your mind whirling, thinking about all the things you have to do the next day. You know you must get to sleep, because if you don't you will feel like a wet rag in the morning, but the more you try, the more sleep evades you. You finally drop off, but morning comes far too quickly, and you get up and drag through the day. Thoroughly exhausted, you fall into bed the next night but the minute your head hits the pillow, you're wide awake, thoughts whirling.

So how do you break the cycle? Sleeping pills are not the answer; they simply knock you out. They don't give your body the type of sleep it requires.

The first thing to realize is that you probably do not need as much sleep as you think you do. Many of the adverse effects of a poor night's sleep are the result of tossing, turning and fretting because you can't get to sleep.

People's sleep requirements differ widely. Some wake refreshed after less than six hours of sleep; others are still tired after ten hours. Some of the great achievers of the world managed on just a few hours a night. Napoleon is reputed to have slept only three or four hours each night (nobody checked up on Wellington!). Churchill was famous for sleeping only a few hours at night and then taking a quick nap during the day. Donald Trump, Maggie Thatcher and Benjamin Franklin were, or are, all short sleepers. You can tell how much sleep you need by how you feel during the day. If you go through the day feeling wide awake, alert and energetic, you're probably getting enough sleep. There is nothing magic in the number eight, although we've all been conditioned to believe we need eight hours of sleep. Listen to your body and experiment a little until you reach the optimum number of hours sleep for yourself.

But remember, being tired and not getting enough sleep are not necessarily the same thing. Tiredness could well be the result of lack of exercise, fresh air or an adequate diet. It is also a side effect of stress. When you are under stress, you may wake up tired even after more than ten hours of sleep. You must learn how to counter the effects of stress by learning to relax. All the things that help you relax will also help you get to sleep and ensure that the sleep you get is refreshing. Because it is the quality of sleep that is important rather than the quantity. An adequate balance between REM sleep (so called because it is accompanied by rapid eye movements) and deep, non-REM sleep is required. Both kinds of sleep are necessary and serve different restorative functions. During deep, non-REM sleep we experience the most physically restorative effects of sleep. During REM sleep we dream, and this is believed to be psychologically beneficial.

The deepest (non-REM) sleep generally occurs when you first go to sleep. You move between non-REM and REM sleep initially but by the time you have slept three hours you will probably have completed your deepest sleep of the night. During the fourth and fifth hours, most of the time you will be experiencing REM sleep and this is when you dream. REM is the shallowest sleep and you are easily woken by noises. That's why you feel as if you were woken up in the middle of a dream.

Sleeping pills help you to fall asleep quickly and to sleep a long time, but they frequently inhibit the deep, non-REM sleep. This means you experience poor quality, non-restorative sleep, and often get up feeling totally washed out even after as much as ten hours sleep. Alcohol helps you get to sleep, but again it can inhibit deep sleep.

Once you are sleeping well, you can manage with less sleep because your sleep is more efficient.

Frequently, it is your state of over-alertness and arousal that prevents you from falling asleep. If you can learn to relax before you go to bed, sleep will come naturally. However, it is no good leaving it until bedtime to relax. It is what happens during the day that affects your sleep. One or two planned sessions of relaxation during the day are important.

If it is at all possible, short naps during the day will promote sound nighttime sleep. Many famous politicians and actors do this to keep operating at top efficiency and to manage with only a few hours sleep at night. At the very least, it takes the anxiety out of a sleepless night if you know you can catch up during the day. And of course with the reduction in anxiety comes sleep. If you are able to take a nap during the day, make it at the same time each day. *Regularity enhances the ability to drop off quickly.*

Before you go to bed, you need to start unwinding. Slow down your mental and physical processes. Set up a series of pre-bed routines, and go through them slowly. With your mind slowly unwinding, drowsiness follows.

Try a few of the following tips:

1. Establish a regular routine before bedtime, and go to bed at the same time each night. Just as you begin to feel hungry around lunchtime, so your body sends signals to your brain that bedtime is approaching, and your temperature drops, your system slows down and you begin to relax. If you keep changing your bedtime, your internal monitor goes haywire. Your brain learns not to relax because it may be called into action at any time.

Have you noticed how difficult it is to get to sleep on Sunday night if you have had two late nights on Friday and Saturday? In even two days your body has started to adjust to a new time.

2. Don't worry about not getting enough sleep. Lack of sleep does not do anything serious to your body. Worry causes you far more problems.

3. If you can't get to sleep after 20 minutes, don't lie fretting about it. Get up and read a while, listen to music or have a glass of milk. It's worth setting up a room as a night-time retreat. You need a comfortable chair, adequate heating, blankets, a reading lamp and, if possible, a facility for making a drink. If everything is at the ready, you don't have to go creeping around finding things and worrying about disturbing the family. After relaxing in your retreat, you'll return to bed and sleep soundly.

Install night lights in the hallway, kitchen and your favorite retreat. Occasionally, you may wake up, start to toss and turn, and have that nasty feeling creep up on you that you aren't going to be able to get back to sleep. However, you still feel drowsy. If you are still drowsy, turning on the light will wake you up completely. So walk along the dimly lit hall to the kitchen and get a glass of milk and a cookie. Sit quietly munching and sipping for a few minutes and perhaps listen to some quiet music, then return to bed.

4. Don't watch violent or disturbing videos or TV programs just before you go to bed.

5. Don't eat a heavy meal just before you go to bed. The meal may make you sleepy, but the quality of your sleep will be poor as your body will be spending a lot of energy digesting the food.

6. Similarly, drinking alcohol will make you sleepy, but the quality of your sleep will be poor. A glass of wine with dinner is fine, but several glasses before you go to bed will not improve your sleep.

7. If you are very hungry, you will have trouble sleeping.

So have a glass of milk and cookies about an hour before you go to bed.

8. Avoid arguments and intensive mental work just before you go to bed.

9. In bed, first stretch and relax your hands one at a time. Then do the same thing with your arms and legs. The relaxation following the tension is transmitted throughout the body.

10. Take an aromatherapy bath with chamomile (2 drops), juniper (3 drops) and marjoram (3 drops) essential oils. Toss in a handful of bath salts, then the oils. You can also pick up a ready mix of essential oils containing a basic relaxation mix from your local health food store. The water should be pleasantly warm, not hot. An over-hot bath is over-stimulating.

11. Read for twenty minutes but not a thriller or a real page-turner.

12. Turn off the light and listen to slow classical music or other soothing music. When you feel drowsy, turn off the tape.

13. Tuck a sleep pillow inside your pillow (see recipe on next page).

14. Meditate during the evening. (Meditation is covered in Chapter 8.)

RECIPE FOR SLEEP PILLOW

Lavender (2 parts)

Lemon Balm (2 parts)

Chamomile (2 parts)

1 part each of the following: rosebuds, marjoram, thyme, sage, rosemary, cinnamon.

Mix the flowers and herbs in a large bowl. Add 3 to 5 drops of lavender, chamomile and marjoram essential oils.

(Essential oils are discussed in Chapter 5.) Sew up the pillow and insert inside your bed pillow.

15. If you have had a poor night's sleep, try to find the time to take a nap at lunchtime. This will not make it more difficult to sleep that night. It will in fact help you to relax and make it easier to fall asleep. Being overly tired makes falling asleep difficult.

Now, it sounds impractical to nip off to bed for a quick snooze at lunchtime. However, you can close your office door, put the phone onto auto, lie back in your chair, put your feet on the waste basket and relax for ten minutes. Kick off your shoes if that is practical and really get into it for a whole ten minutes. You are going to feel very refreshed. If you have a flower on your desk, then spend a few minutes really concentrating on it—enjoy its aroma, admire the texture. As you concentrate on a simple miracle of nature you are pushing out stress-inducing thoughts.

Another trick is to have a picture of the mountains or

the ocean on your wall, and spend ten minutes imagining yourself in the scene enjoying the balmy air and the scent of pines. Sounds flaky, but it works. In ten minutes you can totally refresh your mind. Sleep will come a lot more readily at night.

16. Pay attention to your diet. Too much caffeine and too many sugary foods all inhibit your sleep patterns. Make sure you eat a balanced diet with plenty of fresh vegetables.

17. Coffee, cola and chocolate will all keep you awake. Although here again only you know how much caffeine your body can tolerate before it disturbs your sleep. Also avoid drugs at bedtime that contain caffeine; for example, Exedrin, Migral, Cope, Dexatrim, Anacin.

18. Try a glass of milk about an hour before you go to bed. Mother unquestionably knew best, because milk can be very helpful in inducing sleep. If you don't like milk, then yogurt, brazil nuts, peanuts, pumpkin seeds, sunflower seeds or walnuts will all have the same effect.

19. Listen to your breathing as you lie in bed. Concentrate on each inhalation and exhalation. This drives away intrusive thoughts and before you know it, it's morning.

20. Think pleasant thoughts. If all the worries of the day come pouring in, then try to send your mind away to the beach or a favorite walk.

If You Wake Up in the Night

When you wake up, try to go into a relaxation routine before your mind has time to start rolling again. If you can't drop off after about twenty minutes, get up and do something. Get a glass of warm milk, read for a while and let your body cool off. When you go back to bed the warmth will induce drowsiness. Go through your relaxation routine, and don't get anxious. Promise yourself you'll have an early night tomorrow or a nap during the day. Anxiety produces the chemicals that keep you awake. One night's lost sleep is not going to do you any harm.

You Can Learn to Fall Asleep Easily and Wake Refreshed

The main thing to bear in mind is that sleep is one of the things that can come under your control. It is going to take a little effort and planning, but once you understand your body's needs and learn how to relax, you will be able to drop off to sleep easily and even reduce your sleeping time without it having any ill effects. A short, high-quality, refreshing sleep will leave you well equipped to deal with anything the day can throw at you.

Feeling Tired Frequently Has Nothing to do With Lack of Sleep

If you always feel tired, you probably blame it on lack of sleep, but in fact if you had twelve hours of sleep a night, you could still feel exactly the same way. Exercise and diet have a major effect on your energy level. A poor diet and lack of exercise will leave you feeling listless and edgy no matter how many hours of sleep you get. So make sure you address these two issues if you want to enjoy a healthy sleep pattern.

Regular exercise will promote longer periods of deep, refreshing sleep. However, exercising one to two hours before bedtime will raise your temperature and act as a stimulant, and you will have difficulty in getting to sleep.

Sleeping Well is Just a Question of Habit

We are all creatures of habit. Most of our responses are governed by learned responses imprinted on our subconscious. The most obvious example of this is how hungry you get when lunchtime and dinnertime approach. If you are sleeping poorly, then you have probably programmed yourself to lie awake for a long time before dropping off, or to wake up in the early hours and stare at the ceiling.

Bad habits, fortunately, can be broken. Getting out of a bad habit takes willpower, and acquiring a good one takes some practice, but it can be done. There is no perfect recipe for a good night's sleep. Your lifestyle and your habits are unique. However, if you select some of the suggestions made in this chapter and apply them to your lifestyle, you will be able to solve the problem. What you eat and drink, how much you exercise, how you spend the hour before you go to bed—all influence your sleep patterns. Work out a new routine for yourself, practice your new habits and enjoy deep, refreshing sleep.

FIVE

Aromatherapy

❦❦❦

A romatherapy is a very pleasant and effective way of helping you relax. Just as its name suggests, aromatherapy is the therapeutic use of aroma. The aroma comes from essential oils—highly concentrated plant extracts, which despite their name, are not oily or greasy. By massaging essential oils into the skin, adding them to a warm bath or by inhaling them, stress, tension and insomnia can all be relieved.

The healing properties of essential oils have been acknowledged through the ages but only recently has their contribution to relaxation been truly appreciated. Essential oils are extracted from flowers and plants using a steam distillation process. They can also be squeezed or cold-pressed from fruit. Citrus oils are frequently obtained this way since the essential oils are present in the rind of the fruit. This method is called expression.

These methods differ from those used by the perfume and food industries which use solvents to produce a highly scented concentrate from plants. This is a far cheaper method of extraction but does not produce pure essential oils. For aromatherapy to be effective, you should use only the purest oils—ones that have not been adulterated or diluted. Cheaper, impure oils are not always as effective on a therapeutic level and, in addition, you run the risk of experiencing adverse body reactions to the additives.

Essential oils penetrate the body in two ways: through the nose and the skin. Through our sense of smell, the olfactory nerves pass a message to our brain, and there is a physical and psychological response within a few seconds. For example, the primary cellular unit of the brain is the neuron, which secretes an electrical neurochemical. One of the three neurotransmitter chemicals is serotonin, which is a sedative-like neurochemical produced by the brain to help with relaxation and sleep. The use of essential oils such as lavender and chamomile affect serotonin levels by stimulating the portions of the brain responsible for its production. Essential oils themselves do not cure. They simply stimulate the already active healing, calming and regenerative mechanisms within our body.

Essential oils are also absorbed through the skin. Skin is only about .04 to .08 inch thick on most parts of our body, and about .16 on the palms of our hands and the soles of our feet. Skin is composed of three layers—the outer epidermis, a deep layer called the dermis, which contains the connective tissue that lends skin its strength and suppleness, and the subcutaneous tissue which is responsible for nourishing and insulating us.

Essential oils have the ability to penetrate right into the deep layers of the skin. Once they have passed through the epidermis, they seep into the small capillaries of the dermis, and are carried all around the body in the blood. They are also taken up by the lymph fluid, which bathes every cell in the body.

Aromatic Baths

Aromatic baths are one of the best ways to unwind and relieve tension. They feel especially good at the end of a long day. The warmth of the water, combined with the benefits of the essential oils, melts away muscle tension and relaxes the mind.

When you take a bath, make sure the room is warm and the windows are closed to keep in the vapors. Concentrate on your breathing while you are soaking. Inhale deeply and slowly, letting the pleasant aroma fill your senses, then exhale, pushing out all the negative stresses of the day. Repeat this several times. If you have a tension headache, rub a few drops of lavender essential oil on your temples before soaking in the bath. When leaving the bath, pat your skin lightly, leaving a fine layer of essential oil on your skin's surface for further absorption. For optimum results, take a 15-minute bath.

Hydrotherapy

Hydrotherapy (water healing) in and of itself can be beneficial in relaxing tired muscles and abating stress. When combining it with aromatherapy, you treble the benefits.

The warm water soothes, the relaxing essential oils are inhaled through the nose and are absorbed through the skin. Warm baths (97–101 degrees F.) are the most beneficial. Bath water that is too hot can be counterproductive and leave you looking and feeling like a limp prune.

Since essential oils are not soluble in water, it is best to use them with a carrier—sweet almond, canola or safflower oil. They're great for moisturizing the skin, but they also leave an oil ring in the bath—and do you really need more cleaning? So try bath salts as a carrier—that's the easiest— or Castile unscented liquid soap. You can, of course, just swish the oils around in the bath by themselves, but they tend to evaporate far too quickly.

Then for pure luxury you can use honey or cream as a carrier. The cream is a natural emulsifier and great for dry skin. Just think about driving home through rush hour traffic in anticipation of a warm, scented bath laced with cream. Pure decadence beckons. Cleopatra swore by it.

If you're not into decadence, then bergamot (3 drops), cedarwood (2 drops) and lavender (3 drops), or alternatively, orange (2 drops), lavender (3 drops) and patchouli (2 drops) swished around in the water with a handful of bath salts is fine.

But I Don't Have Time for a Bath

So how about trying a footbath? Maurice Messegué, a famous French herbalist and natural healer, perfected the art of healing footbaths. Herbs were added to water, and the patient absorbed the benefits of the oils through the skin of the feet, and these spread quickly through the body.

If you don't believe this, cut a garlic clove in half, put it on the sole of your foot, then breathe on your partner an hour later.

To prepare a footbath, you need a plastic bowl big enough to fit both feet comfortably, a towel, some essential oils and about 10 to 15 minutes. You can do it while reading reports (at home—not at work), checking the kids' homework, watching TV or reading a novel. Half fill the bowl with warm water, and away you go. A rectangular bowl (available from most hardware stores) is more practical than a round one. Your feet fit easily and you don't need such a large bowl.

If you use rosemary (3 drops) and peppermint (2 drops) essential oils, the footbath will have an uplifting, stimulating effect on your emotions as well as a rejuvenating effect on your feet. Alternatively, rosemary (2 drops), sage (2 drops) and tea tree (1 drop) can have the same effect.

Would you believe a cold footbath with essential oils (4 drops lavender, 2 drops peppermint) is also good for tension headaches? Soaking your feet in cold water draws blood from your head, bringing immediate relief. Sit comfortably with both feet immersed for about 15 minutes. Concentrate on breathing slowly and relaxing.

Eye Pillows

For mild eyestrain and headaches, try an eye pillow. You can keep them in your desk drawer or beside your bed. Eye pillows are rectangular in shape and are filled with lentils, rice, oats or other grains. The grain gives them weight and also helps mold them to your eyes with a pleasant, gentle pressure. To make an eye pillow you need:

Flaxseed—1 cup; lavender—1 cup; and lavender essential oil—3-5 drops. Put into a rectangle of silk or cotton large enough to cover the eyes comfortably and sew opening.

Vaporizers

Using a vaporizer is a great way to permeate the atmosphere with the delightful aromas of pure essential oils. As the oils evaporate, our sensitive olfactory nerves transmit the aroma to the brain. The tranquilizing effect on our mind and body starts within minutes. You need a ceramic vaporizer and a few drops of your favorite oil or a combination of oils. Put about six drops of the chosen oil in a shallow dish filled with water. Light the small candle under the dish. The heat from the candle slowly evaporates the water and oils into the surrounding air.

Business Trips

You probably already know the trick of spreading a few personal belongings in your hotel room as soon as you arrive to make it feel more like home and reduce the stress induced by strange places. A photo of your partner, kids or dog, a toothbrush and toiletries, and a paperback novel all help. Now try taking along a vaporizer and your favorite essential oils; the ones you use at home. The soothing vapor permeating the room will have a wonderfully relaxing effect.

WHICH OILS TO SELECT

If you go to an Aromatherapist, they will select the oils they feel will be most beneficial to you. However, since initially you may not have time to visit one, here are a few anti-stress essential oil combinations.

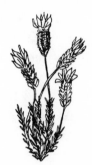

6 drops lavender essential oil
1 drop sandalwood essential oil
OR
1 drop basil essential oil
2 drops juniper essential oil
2 drops lavender essential oil
1 drop ylang-ylang essential oil

Note: Everyone reacts to aromas in slightly different ways. Experiment to find which of the blends make you feel good. (A word of caution: do not increase the amount of oil, rather change blends as overdoing a fragrance can be counter-productive.)

A Few More Ideas for Using Essential Oils

• Put a drop of lavender on a tissue and tuck it in the air vent in the car.

• Hook up a diffuser in the work area. Inhalation of essential oils during the day is an easy way to enjoy the benefits of aromatherapy.

TO RELIEVE STRESS
all of the following are good:

Bergamot, cedarwood, chamomile, geranium, lavender, marjoram, rose otto, sandalwood, ylang-ylang, frankincense, myrrh and neroli.

FOR A PICK-ME-UP:

Basil, lemon, rosemary, sage and pine.

FOR MEDITATION:

Frankincense, and myrrh. (A little gold might help relieve your stress too.) You will also find pre-mixed massage oil blends at your local health food store or pharmacist.

• Simply inhale from a tissue to which you have applied a few drops of essential oil.

• Take a facecloth and essential oils to work in your handbag or briefcase. Then at lunchtime or whenever you pop to the restroom, run hot water over the facecloth, add a drop of essential oil, squeeze out excess moisture, then hold it to your face and breathe deeply. Adding lavender (1 drop) and neroli (2 drops) will help you to relax. Or use lemon (1 drop) and rosemary (2 drops) to sharpen your mind.

• Another way to make the office or your home smell good, and to enhance the air of relaxation, is a room mister.

Simply add 10-12 drops of lavender and marjoram essential oils to 4 ounces distilled water in a spray bottle. Use a blue or amber glass bottle or stainless steel spray can.

Don't use a plastic container for essential oils. Shake well before each use because oil and water do not mix naturally. The calming effects of lavender and marjoram will permeate the office and lighten up the most harassing day.

Essential Oil Ratings

Essential oils are rated for their volatility and categorized into Top, Middle and Base Notes. Top Notes vaporize quickly and require most care in storage since they are the most volatile. Base Notes are the slowest to evaporate. The most balanced and lasting aromatherapy blends are the ones that include Top, Middle and Base Notes.

Storing Oils

Store essential oils in glass containers, preferably amber or blue. Keep them in a refrigerator or a cool, dark place. *Keep out of the reach of children.*

Massage

Massage, particularly aromatherapy massage, is a great way to reduce stress. An aromatherapy massage combines the relaxing properties of essential oils with the benefits of touch and therapeutic massage. Muscles are encouraged to relax with every massage stroke, while essential oils with their healing properties are absorbed through the skin's surface. Massage stimulates the circulation of blood to the surface of the skin, thereby increasing the absorption of oils into your body.

Essential oils will not be absorbed well when the body is eliminating—when sweating through anxiety or heat, for instance, or after exercise. Their efficiency in penetration can also be impeded by a large amount of subcutaneous fat or poor circulation.

A good massage takes practice and a few developed skills. Ideally, going to a professional—taking along the mix of oils you prefer—is the way to go. If you go to an Aromatherapist, they will ask you about medical history, allergies, physical condition, lifestyle, etc., and then prepare a blend of oils suited to your needs.

> Essential oils in the pure state are too highly concentrated to be used directly on the skin. They should be diluted in a base or carrier oil.

However, if you can't get to a professional, you can enjoy massage at home if you can convince your partner to participate. Or you can always give yourself a mini-massage; a 2-minute massage with your favorite essential oil after your shower in the morning can be a great way to start the day. Tips on how to give a massage and how to mix massage oils can be found in the Appendix.

Essential Oils

The following essential oils are all good for combating stress. They are listed to provide you with basic information to get you started. But do bear in mind that you can always go to your local health food store, pharmacy, or any other good store where they sell essential oils to get additional advice. My experience has been that they are delighted to help beginners.

All essential oils are anti-bacterial, anti-viral and anti-septic. *Do not use essential oils directly on the skin without first diluting them with a carrier oil.* The exception to this is lavender and tea tree which can be applied directly to small areas.

To dilute essential oils with a carrier oil, pour 10 ml* sweet almond (or other carrier oil) in a glass dish, then add 5 drops of your selected essential oils. The rule of thumb is half as many drops of essential oil to the number of ml in the carrier oil. The carrier oil need not be exact, but it is important to measure essential oils carefully. Mix them together and pour into a bath, or leave in the dish for massage.

The Top, Middle and Base Notes indicate their volatility. Top Notes vaporize most quickly and Base Notes are the slowest to evaporate. Balance your blends by including Top, Middle and Base Notes.

* **Note:** One milliliter (ml) = 1 cubic centimeter (cc); 1 cc = 20 drops; 5 cc = 1 teaspoon = 100 drops.

BASIL (Ocimum basilicum)   *Top Note*
Basil is distilled from the herb. Basil's rich peppery-anise aroma refreshes overworked minds and bodies. An ideal pick-me-up when you are feeling tired. Blends well with bergamot, geranium and lavender. Do not use during pregnancy.

BERGAMOT (Citrus Bergamia)   *Top Note*
Bergamot is an uplifting oil, helping disperse anxiety and relieve stress. Bergamot is pressed from the fresh peel of a

small orange first grown in Northern Italy. Bergamot blends well with cypress, jasmine, lavender and neroli. Bergamot should not be used if you are going out in the sun since it increases the skin's photosensitivity.

CHAMOMILE (Anthemis nobilis; Matricaria chamomilla; Oremenis mixta)   *Middle Note*

Chamomile is a gentle essential oil which has a calming, soothing effect on both the body and the mind. It both relieves stress and helps dispel insomnia. It is distilled from the chamomile flower. It blends well with geranium, lavender, patchouli and rose otto. In Tudor times, poets waxed lyrical while reclining on chamomile-perfumed turf.

CEDARWOOD (Juniperus virginiana)   *Base Note*

One of the oldest essential oils, cedarwood relieves deep-down stress and chronic anxiety. It blends well with bergamot, cypress, jasmine, juniper, neroli and rosemary. Extracted from the wood of Juniperus Virginiana in the U.S., its fragrance is that of a fresh-cut tree. It is good to use at the beginning of the weekend or the beginning of your vacation to put you in the right frame of mind to enjoy them. Use bergamot, lavender and cedarwood as a "beginning of weekend" mix. And, incidentally, cedarwood used in conjunction with rosemary can also promote hair growth!

CLARY SAGE (Salvia sclarea)   *Top Note*

Distilled from flowers, clary sage helps relax, uplift you and dispel depressed thinking. It also helps reduce high blood pressure. It blends well with cedarwood, citrus oils, frankincense, geranium, jasmine, juniper, lavender and sandalwood.

FRANKINCENSE (Boswellia carterii)   *Base Note*

Frankincense is collected from the sweet-smelling resin shed by Boswellia carterii, small trees grown in Saudi Arabia and Somaliland. Very relaxing; it has a calming effect on the mind and emotions. It is also a useful aid to meditation. Blends well with basil, black pepper, citrus oils, geranium, lavender, pine and sandalwood. One of the ancient world's most highly prized substances.

GERANIUM (Pelargonium graveolens)   *Middle Note*

Distilled from the green parts of the geranium. Geranium helps balance mood swings and relieves tension. Blends well with nearly all oils, especially basil, citrus oils and rose otto.

LAVENDER (Lavendula angustifolia)   *Middle Note*

Lavender is distilled from silvery lilac spikes of the well known shrub. Lavender is the most versatile of all the essential oils. It relieves the symptoms of anxiety, stress and insomnia. A few drops on the pillow or in a warm bath encourages sleep. Blends well with most oils, especially citrus oils, clary sage, patchouli, pine and rosemary. Unlike other oils, it can be applied directly to the skin on a small area—and is in fact good for minor burns and insect bites. Its properties of burn healing were discovered by Dr. Gattefossé, one of the founding fathers of aromatherapy, when he severely burned his hand in his laboratory and plunged his hand accidentally into a bowl of lavender essential oil. The pain stopped and his hand healed quickly afterwards. For severe burns I would strongly recommend a doctor, but for minor ones, cool the burn under running cold water, then apply lavender oil and cover with gauze.

LEMON (Citrus limonum) *Top Note*

Lemon essential oil is pressed from the outer skin of the fruit. The refreshing aroma of lemon is a good pick-me-up after a tiring day. Blends well with lavender and neroli. Do not use out in the sun since it increases the skin's photo-sensitivity.

MARJORAM (Origanum majorana) *Middle Note*

Marjoram is distilled from the flowering tips of the herb. It has a sedative effect, providing comfort when you are feeling low. It is not suitable for heavy depression. Helps with insomnia when blended with orange. Blends well with lavender, bergamot and rosemary.

MYRRH (Commiphora myrrha) *Base Note*

Myrrh is distilled from a gum resin. It is fortifying for the mind. Provides courage and support for demanding physical and emotional situations. They say no soldier of Ancient Greece went into battle without some myrrh in his pouch. So it sounds just right before you go to your next meeting. Also a good aid to meditation. Blends well with camphor and lavender. Do not use during pregnancy.

NEROLI (Citrus aurantium, amara) *Middle to Base Note*

Distilled from the flowers of the Seville orange, it has a beautiful perfume when diluted. Reduces anxiety and stress, keeps you calm and stops you worrying so much.

Also helps with insomnia. Blends well with benzoin, clary sage, geranium and lavender.

PINE (Pinus Sylvestris) *Middle Note*
Distilled from the needles and cones of several species of conifer. The crisp, exhilarating fragrance of pine helps troubled minds relax. Also good for muscular aches and pains. It has a stimulating effect on the circulation and helps you get more oxygen. Blends well with cedarwood, lavender, petitgrain and rosemary.

ROSEMARY (Rosmarinus officinalis) *Middle Note*
Distilled from the herb, rosemary essential oil has a brisk, clear and penetrating herbal aroma. It has a strong effect on the nervous system, acting as a brain stimulant to heighten sensory perception and memory. Blends well with basil, cedarwood, citrus oils, frankincense, lavender and peppermint. Not to be used if you are suffering from high blood pressure or epilepsy.

ROSE OTTO (Rosa damascena) *Base to Middle Note*
Rose otto has a beautiful aroma, and generally only one drop is needed for most purposes. It nurtures you and restores confidence and helps encourage emotional stability. Also very helpful with insomnia. Blends well with bergamot, clary sage, geranium, jasmine, patchouli and sandalwood.

SANDALWOOD (Santalum album) *Base Note*
Sandalwood oil is extracted from the innermost heartwood of a slow growing evergreen from the Indian mountains of

Mysore. The tree is conserved, and only trees at the end of their lifespan are used. The oil is obtained by steam distillation. Helps relieve nervous tension, depression and insomnia. Has a stabilizing influence. Helps with meditation. Blends well with benzoin, black pepper, cypress, frankincense, neroli and ylang-ylang.

YLANG-YLANG (Cananga odorata)   *Middle to Base Note*

Ylang-ylang essential oil is distilled from an exotic tropical flower. Its exotic aroma relaxes stressful states. It is very soothing and pacifying. Has a settling effect on rapid heartbeat. Good for insomnia. Blends well with most oils, especially jasmine and sandalwood. Excessive use may cause nausea and headaches.

NOTE:

Rose otto, sandalwood, and ylang-ylang all have aphrodisiac qualities.

Marjoram is an anti-aphrodisiac.

So, if either of these conditions is contributing to your stress level, add a few drops to the potion.

For further information on aromatherapy, refer to the following books.

Practical Aromatherapy by Shirley Price. Published by Thorsons.

Essential Aromatherapy by Susan Worwood. Published by New World Library.

Aromatherapy Secrets by Nerys Purchon. Published by Hodder & Stoughton.

Aromatherapy and Massage by Christine Wildwood. Published by Thorsons.

The Fragrant Art of Aromatherapy. Published by Lansdowne Publishing.

SIX

Diet and Nutrition

Another essential component of your anti-stress campaign is a healthy diet. Cut down on caffeine, alcohol, red meat and colas. Make sure your diet is balanced and full of nutritious food. Forget junk food and takeouts. Keep slim by exercising and eating fresh, healthy food, not by taking pills.

Why do you need to bother about your diet when your real problem is stress? It is very simple. If you are not eating correctly, you are doubling up the effect of each stressful situation. The brain is very sensitive. When essential proteins, fatty acids, vitamins and minerals are not sufficiently available, brain cells degenerate rapidly, causing a deteriorating emotional and intellectual capacity. If food intake is inadequate, the brain, like the body, must draw on reserves to function. Eventually the reserves are depleted and your ability to deal with stress is severely impaired.

Lack of correct nourishment also inflicts physical stress on the body, and this inevitably causes some form of physical reaction. The reaction differs from person to person but tends to hit wherever your particular weakness lies. When you are under heavy mental stress at the same time, then the reaction will in all probability be in the adrenal glands. So your poor adrenal glands that are already pumping overtime dealing with the latest fight or flight office crisis have a physical problem to deal with as well. The result is chronic fatigue, headaches, insomnia and all those other nasty side effects of stress.

It isn't difficult to eat properly. You can eat well, enjoy the food and find it easier to keep your weight under control. Your body needs a balanced level of body building proteins, energy giving fats and carbohydrates, dietary fiber and the full range of vitamins and minerals. Unless you are already on a well-balanced diet, you probably need to cut down on animal fats, reduce your intake of protein, cut out processed and refined foods and step up on fruits, vegetables and whole grain cereals.

The gist of all the information being generated by the American Heart Association, and other medical bodies, is that you need to reduce by half your intake of calories from fat and animal protein, and to at least double your intake of calories from vegetables, fruits, whole grains and legumes.

Our body prefers to get its energy from carbohydrates. Fats are its second choice. So to keep your energy level up, you need carbohydrates in your diet. There are two types of carbohydrates—"good" or complex carbohydrates and "bad" or refined carbohydrates.

Complex carbohydrates consist of plant foods in their original state. They are still whole and have not been depleted by processing or manufacturing. Stone ground milling of grain into flour or oats is okay, because the flour and oats retain most of the original fiber and nutrients.

Refined carbohydrates start out as wheat, sugar or rice, but during processing they are stripped of almost all the fiber and other nutrients. White flour, white sugar, and white rice are mostly empty calories. White rice isn't quite as bad as the flour and sugar, but brown rice is better.

You do still get fast energy from refined carbohydrates but, because the cell walls have been destroyed by milling, the starches and sugars are rapidly released and transformed into glucose which pours into the bloodstream in a sudden rush. The flood of glucose overwhelms the ability of the pancreas to secrete insulin. Instead of turning the surplus glucose into glycogen, to be stored in the liver and muscles for future use, the rush of glucose simply drives up the blood sugar level. You soon use this up and, without glycogen reserves to draw on, the blood sugar level then plummets. The result is low blood sugar, leaving you drained of energy.

By contrast, complex carbohydrates are composed of living cells each enclosed by a cellulose wall. It takes time for the body to break down the cellulose, which means the complex carbohydrates are released at a steady rate. The muscles now have a slow-burning fuel, and the roller coaster effect of dropping blood sugar does not occur. The discarded cellulose supplies the digestive system with the fiber it needs to function well.

The following is a selection of complex carbohydrates.

FRUITS

Apples, apricots, avocados, bananas, cherries, grapes, melons, papayas, peaches, pineapples, raisins

LEGUMES

Beans, peas

TUBERS OR ROOT VEGETABLES

Beets, carrots, parsnips, potatoes, sweet potatoes, turnips, yams

VEGETABLES

Cucumbers, pumpkin, squash

WHOLE GRAINS

Barley, whole-grain bread, whole-wheat flour, corn, muesli, oatmeal, whole-grain pasta, brown rice, shredded wheat, sunflower seeds

NUTS

Peanuts, walnuts, cashew nuts, etc.

Following are some of the refined carbohydrates to avoid:

Candy, chocolate, white flour, white sugar, pies, pastries, ice cream, cakes, cookies.

The body is good at conserving sodium and poor at conserving potassium. So you need a high potassium, low sodium diet. In their natural state, most fruits and vegetables are high in potassium and low in sodium.

Food processing tends to reverse the situation and in addition strips the food of most of its vitamins. If you are always eating processed foods, rather than foods in their natural state—such as salads and fresh fruit—then you will elevate your sodium level (which can lead to high blood pressure) and also suffer from vitamin deficiency.

Make sure you include adequate fiber in your diet. The skins of vegetables and fruit are a good source. It is also present in grains, breads, cereals, seeds and nuts. Animal foods (beef, lamb, pork, etc.) do not provide dietary fiber. Monounsaturated fats found in olive oil and many nuts help keep cholesterol at a low level in the body.

Include food rich in Vitamin B and C in your diet since these are used up quickly by the body. Vitamin B is found in yeast, wheat germ, fish and soy beans. Vitamin C in citrus fruits, strawberries, melons, grapes, asparagus, broccoli, potatoes with skin and cabbage.

Make sure you include iron-rich food in your diet. Shellfish (especially mussels), sardines, lean red meat, green leafy vegetables, beets, chickpeas, kidney beans and dried fruit are all good sources of iron. If you are an endurance athlete, vegetarian, menstruating woman or on a limited food intake diet, your body has an increased need for iron.

Of the two types of iron, haem iron, found in red meat, is well absorbed by the body whereas your body has more trouble absorbing non-haem iron, present in vegetables and plants. So eat foods rich in Vitamin C (citrus fruit, red and green peppers) with meals to enhance the absorption of iron, and reduce your intake of tea, coffee and cola. Drinking tea, coffee and cola with your meals hinders iron absorption.

Drink plenty of spring water daily. Eight glasses is the recommended amount. If eight glasses sounds daunting, try carrying around a 1.5 litre container of water.

Table A, page 57, illustrates the major food groups. If you include something from each group every day, you will

TABLE A
A BALANCED DIET

GROUP 1 **Breads and Cereals**
Whole-grain bread, rice and pasta, oatmeal,
cereals (not the sugary sort)

GROUP 2 **Vegetables and Fruits**
All fruits and vegetables
Citrus, tropical and berry fruits, tomatoes—for
Vitamin C
Spinach, broccoli, swiss chard, carrots, pumpkin,
apricots, canteloupe—for Vitamin A

GROUP 3 **Meats, beans, nuts, etc.**
Beef, lamb, pork, poultry, eggs, fish, dried peas
and beans, lentils, nuts

GROUP 4 **Milk Products**
Milk, yoghurt, cheese, butter, cream

GROUP 5 **Oils**
Olive oil, soya oil, saffola oil

obtain all the vitamins, minerals and nutrients you need.

Remember, you need to reduce by half your intake of calories from fat and meat in Groups 3 and 4. Cheese, cream, ice cream and sausages are all loaded with fat. And fat lurks in chocolate and pastry.

Double up your intake of calories from Groups 1 and 2—vegetables, fruits, whole-grain bread. The great thing about Groups 1 and 2 (the complex carbohydrates) is that they fill you up without filling you out.

Cut down on meat and eat more fish and vegetable sources of protein (nuts, peas, beans and lentils).

Note the lack of items like cake, candy, soft drinks, ice cream and cookies. This doesn't mean you shouldn't eat them. Just make sure they are occasional treats rather than a mainstay of your diet. Similarly, takeout food once a week will not do you too much harm, but a steady diet of greasy fries and sugary hamburger buns will.

To ensure a balanced diet, select foods from each of the five food groups in Table A, in the proportions illustrated below. Note the recommended percentages are 10% fat, 15% protein and 70% complex carbohydrates, versus the average diet currently consumed which is 40-45% fat, 10-15% protein, and 40-45% carbohydrates (mostly refined). The 5% sin food is my contribution to medical statistics.

RECOMMENDED PROPORTIONS IN A DAILY DIET

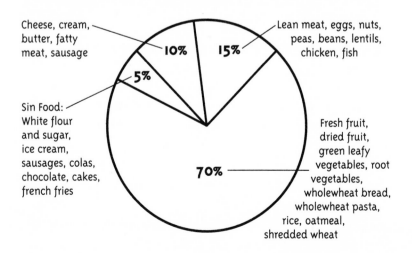

This is just a brief summary of some of the things you can do to start fueling your body correctly so that it can counteract stress. It is by no means a complete picture of all the things you need to know about correct nutrition. My aim is simply to remind you of some of the things you may well be ignoring if you are under pressure at work. I would encourage you to read more on the subject from one of the following books:

The New Pritiken Program by Robert Pritiken. Published by Simon & Schuster, 1990.

Good Housekeeping Healthy Eating by Susana Tee. Published by Ebury Press.

Let's Eat Right to Keep Fit by Adele Davis. The New American Library, 1970.

Or talk to a dietitian or your family doctor.

One last thought. If you get hungry towards the end of the day, and you're feeling empty and tired when a stressful situation occurs, your body is not ready to cope. So in mid-afternoon, drink some fruit juice, eat a piece of fruit, a fat-free granola bar, a couple of whole-grain fig bars or some sunflower seeds.

Listen to your body and treat it right.

SEVEN

Reflexology

ꕥꕥ

How often do you pay attention to your feet? Probably not a lot. The only time you remember them is when they are killing you at the end of a long day, or when you're debating whether you can afford a pair of Bally shoes.

However, feet are quite remarkable. Leonardo da Vinci called the foot "a masterpiece of engineering." They take the entire weight of your body in a very small area. They are your primary link with the earth. They are used constantly all day in one way or another and are frequently scrunched into shoes designed more for fashion than comfort.

Do you remember all those horror stories about Chinese women having their feet bound? A practice that fortunately died out long ago. That's because a woman's foot was regarded as the ultimate sex symbol. Binding the feet stunted growth and made them more desirable. What has this got to do with stress? Nothing. But you must admit regarding feet as the ultimate sex symbol puts them in a new light.

Your feet are one of the most sensitive areas of your body and have an important role to play in your health and well-being. The thousands of nerve endings in your feet have a vital connection with all parts of the body.

Reflexology is a form of therapeutic foot massage that can reduce stress and promote relaxation. Working on the principle that there are reflex areas on the feet that correspond with all the different parts of the body, reflexologists use specific pressure techniques to restore and maintain good health. It is a thoroughly uncomplicated technique which has proved to be very effective.

Although there is no satisfactory scientific explanation as to why massaging a pressure point in your foot can, for example, cure a headache, the fact is it works. Certainly both the Chinese and the Egyptians have been practicing it successfully for several thousand years. Since modern Western medicine has only been around for a few hundred years, and our current drug-based medicine less than a hundred, it is worth giving it a try.

A general massage of the feet is extremely pleasant and relaxing—in fact, a few people have been known to drop off to sleep during a reflexology treatment. Then, as the reflexologist works on the pressure points of your foot and discovers areas of tension in the corresponding area of your body, stress can be dispelled by more intense massage. The areas might be tight muscles in the shoulders and neck, and an adrenal gland oversensitized by prolonged stress.

An overall foot massage at bedtime is also excellent for

combating insomnia. The overall foot massage induces a relaxed state which can then be followed by gentle stroking, particularly over the top of the foot. This, of course, is where a cooperative partner comes in handy, although you can sit in bed and massage your own feet.

Through the diagnosis obtained by massaging your feet, a reflexologist can detect health problems early on, and treatment can be given to prevent serious symptoms from developing. By massaging your feet, which in itself is extremely relaxing, the reflexologist can detect stress points such as your adrenal glands and head, and help dispel the tension and discomforts produced by stress.

Reflexology is a holistic healing art form which falls into the realm of alternative medicine. As with most practices in this category, disease is approached from the understanding of man as a complex organism comprised of body, mind and spirit. The object of holistic treatment is to induce a state of balance and harmony throughout the entire organism.

A word about "alternative medicine." Currently it covers anything which does not fall into the mainstream of orthodox Western medicine. A more accurate title would be "complementary" medicine. Reflexology can be a helpful adjunct to current medical practice. Since it addresses the whole person—body, mind and spirit—it can be particularly helpful in dealing with stress-related problems.

In traditional Eastern medical systems—notably the Chinese healing system and the Indian Ayurvedic system—it has long been established that health is based on the harmonious flow of energies. Both zone therapy and meridian therapy are based on the premise that energy channels, or

ENERGY CHANNELS

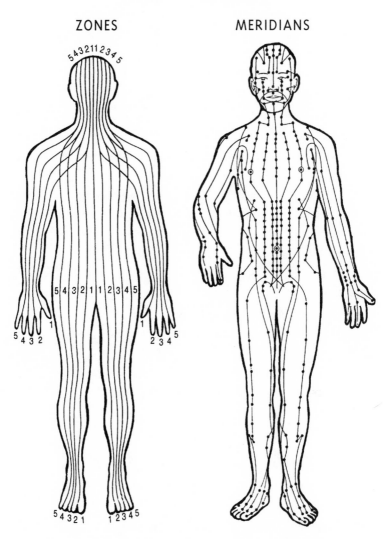

ZONES   MERIDIANS

pathways, traverse the body, linking organs and body parts. The effectiveness of reflexology is believed to be the result of stimulating and revitalizing this energy flow.

The holistic health philosophy considers the human body as a dynamic energy system in a constant state of change. Because we cannot see energy with the naked eye, we find it hard to comprehend. In Chinese and Indian Ayurvedic medicine, health is seen as the fluent and harmonious movement of energies at subtle levels.

The Indian yogis call it prana, sakia-tundra or ki to the Japanese, Shinto and ch'i to the Chinese. The nearest translation to us would probably be vital energy or life force. According to Eastern tradition, this energy permeates every living cell and tissue of our body, and it has clearly distinct and established pathways and definite direction of flow, as well defined as any other circulation such as blood and the vascular system.

In a healthy person, under normal circumstances, the life force, ch'i, flows evenly, maintaining a balance between the vigorous yang and restraining yin elements. If either yang or yin becomes too dominant, the body's harmony is jeopardized.

For the reflexologist there are ten channels beginning (or ending) in the toes and extending to the fingers and to the top of the head. Each channel relates to a zone of the body and to the organs in that zone. For example, the big toe relates to the head.

Reflexology in Relation to Acupuncture

For thousands of years the Chinese have practiced acupuncture. This involves inserting needles into certain areas of the body known as acupuncture points. These points are

THE THEORY OF YIN AND YANG

The ancient Chinese believed that a life force flows along meridians which correspond to different parts of the body. The activating force behind ch'i is the constant movement of energy between two poles or extremes known as yin and yang. These correspond to our ideas of positive and negative, or male and female, forces. In order to be healthy and enjoy a sense of well-being, the yin and yang forces must be perfectly balanced.

situated on lines known as meridian, or energy, lines distributed throughout the body.

By placing a needle at a certain point, energy within a meridian can be redistributed which results in a correction of an ailment associated with this meridian. Often a needle is inserted in an area quite distant from the part of the body requiring treatment, but it is effective because it is linked to that part of the body by the meridian line.

Reflexology is based on similar lines to acupuncture in that there are energy lines linking the feet to various parts of the body, and the whole body can be worked on by working on the reflex areas in the feet. The energy lines of reflexology are not exactly the same as acupuncture meridian lines, but the similarities are there. And, of course, a very fundamental difference is that in acupuncture needles are used. In reflexology, only massage with the hands is used.

Visiting a Reflexologist

First, how do you find a reflexologist? Try at your local health food store; they generally have listings; or you may find them in the directory under therapeutic massage. Another way to find them is through your local doctor. Ask his or her opinion. If she's open minded, she may have a list of reputable people who practice alternative medicine. When you visit a reflexologist, they first ask you about yourself and any problems you are having. Then they have you remove your stockings or socks, and shoes, and get up on a massage table. Alternatively, they may simply ask you to sit in a chair. They cover you with warm towels and wrap one of your feet in a warm towel.

Using massage oil, they gently massage your entire foot, then start to work their way through the terminals of energy on each foot, applying pressure. The object is to find energy blocks and to get rid of them by specialized massaging techniques. Reflexologists believe the overall massage of the feet promotes the body's natural self-healing properties and is a good preventative health measure.

Certainly, a foot massage relaxes the whole body and mind and can leave you in a calm, relaxed state. At the end of an hour's massage, your feet feel tingly and invigorated. The reflexologist recommends that you drink plenty of water after a session to facilitate the flushing of toxins released by the massage.

Foot massage once a month, with the right blend of essential oils, can be surprisingly relaxing. A good reflexologist will welcome using your own favorite blend of oils.

A few people I have spoken to did not enjoy their reflexology treatment. They maintained that when the reflexologist applied pressure on their foot corresponding to an area in their body where they were having trouble, it hurt. For example, if they suffered from asthma the area on their foot corresponding to their chest hurt when massaged. They did not return for another session. Other people mentioned discomfort the first time they visited when the reflexologist located a problem area, but gradually lessening discomfort on subsequent visits both on their foot and with the complaint the reflexologist was treating. Personally, I experienced no problems with my first visit, or subsequent visit, and found it both relaxing and intriguing. It still seems like black magic to me that they can massage my foot and detect I have a lower back problem. If you do go, and by any chance they detect a problem, then go to your doctor and let him or her check it for you. All the remedies for stress suggested in this book should be coupled with regular physical checkups with your doctor.

You can, of course, massage your own feet, although without a great deal of study, you are not going to be able to duplicate the reflexologist's skills. However, as an emergency measure, or for general relaxation, it can be beneficial. The Appendix provides the basics of the techniques.

For further information on reflexology, refer to:

The Art of Reflexology by Inge Dougans with Suzanne Ellis, published by Barnes & Noble.

The Reflexology Manual by Pauline Wills, published by Healing Arts Press, 1995.

EIGHT

Meditation

One of the surest ways to combat stress is by meditation. Nothing else is quite as effective in initiating the relaxation response. Twenty minutes in the morning and in the evening can make a major change to your life. The methods we have talked about so far will lead to a more relaxed state of mind, but meditation can take you a step further. Research has shown that a number of physiological changes take place during meditation. Tension and stress are reduced but in addition meditation has been found to produce a heightened alertness and ability to concentrate. Behavior patterns involving things like smoking and overeating can be improved or controlled by meditation. And high blood pressure, one of the results of stress, can be substantially improved by successful meditation.

Meditation is basically stilling the mind and getting rid of all the whirling thoughts and frustrating residues of the day's traumas. Meditation diverts the conscious mind from everyday thought processes and induces a state of peacefulness and well-being.

However, learning to meditate takes application. You can take classes which generally last for one and a half to two hours per day for four days, read meditation methods from a book, or write away for a written do-it-yourself meditation kit. Learning the technique is very simple; applying it takes longer. Some people can do it immediately. Others take as long as six months to start to enjoy the full benefits of meditation. However, even during the learning stages, you are beginning to reduce stress.

Most people experience a sense of inner calm and feel very relaxed after regularly practicing mediation. You may also feel refreshed, a sense of pleasure, and a general sense of well-being. You may even, if you are one of the lucky minority, feel ecstatic. However, according to medical research, even people who feel none of these sensations still enjoy the physiological benefits: lower blood pressure, slower heart and respiratory rates. It would appear that meditation encourages the body to counteract the "fight or flight" response induced by stress.

Many forms of meditation are taught in courses and books. The predominant one is Transcendental Meditation (TM). To transcend literally means "to go beyond." In TM you learn to go beyond the noise of your whirling thoughts to a region of peace and tranquillity. Maharishi Mahesh Yogi, who brought his system of Transcendental Meditation to the west in the '60s, defines the state achieved in meditation as "restful alertness," the meditator is alert but not thinking about anything—ideally, not thinking at all. This state of restful alertness is pleasant in itself, but what really matters is that the deep rest provided by meditation undoes the harmful effects of stress.

As with all the forms of relaxation we have talked about so far, different methods of learning meditation suit different people. Some will enjoy and benefit from the spiritual approach; others will prefer a more pragmatic approach. For the pragmatists, books that cover meditation include:

Stress by Leon Chaitow in the Thorson's Health Series. Published by Harper Collins.

The Relaxation Response by Herbert Benson, M.D. Published by Collins.

The Joy of Meditating. A Beginner's Guide to the Art of Meditation by Salle Merrill Redfield. Published by Warner Books.

Another approach is *Meditation Pure & Simple* by Dr. Ian Gawler Hill of Content Publishing.

However, the easy approach is to go to a large bookstore and ask for a recommendation, then browse the shelf.

If you are under extreme stress, you may find it difficult to meditate. In this case, you should precede meditation with breathing exercises to reduce your stress level, or with a warm bath to help you relax. Another approach would be to write down the things that are worrying you and then to do a few neutral chores around the house. If you are in a highly charged stressful state, this should bring you down from fifth gear to fourth. Now you are ready to meditate. After a few sessions approaching meditation this way, you should be able to dispense with these preliminaries.

You may frequently find during meditation that your

thoughts continue to intrude, preventing you from achieving peace of mind. Don't worry about this. By sitting and letting the thoughts whirl, you are getting them out of your system. Initially, you may only be able to achieve a few moments of perfect peace and relaxation during your 20-minute session but if you persevere this will grow longer and longer.

Since in this age of the instant fix we all expect immediate results, you will probably become frustrated if you don't immediately float off to a peaceful place for twenty minutes twice a day. Persevere. It is worth it. As you practice you are ridding yourself of all the stresses and strains of the day. It may not seem that way if thoughts keep intruding, but you are on the path to stress reduction. Meditation experience increases with repetition. To organize your life and discipline yourself to do it twice a day will take some effort. But you will find once it becomes part of your daily routine you will look forward to the oasis of calm and regeneration the period of meditation brings.

One way to find the time is to spend twenty minutes in your car at lunchtime. Not while you're driving of course! Or if it's possible to lock the office door, take twenty minutes during the lunch break. A cup of coffee and a sandwich will be a good cover.

Get up twenty minutes earlier each morning. A gruesome thought. But you probably did it in order to go out jogging when you were serious about losing weight. The relaxation you will ultimately enjoy as a result of meditation will help you sleep more deeply and make up for the lost twenty minutes.

It is better to do it earlier in the evening rather than just before you go to bed because you may find yourself totally refreshed by meditation with all your tiredness gone. So do it early and enjoy a better quality of life for the remainder of the evening.

One caution about meditating for twenty minutes when you first get home. If you live alone, or your partner arrives home a lot later than you, it will be okay. However, if you have a housebound partner, who has been eagerly awaiting your return, saying, "Hi, honey, good to see you, now I must go and meditate for twenty minutes," won't go over in a big way. Also if your partner likes to come home and spend the first half hour telling you about his or her traumas of the day, it won't be popular. If these situations apply, then think about spending an extra twenty minutes in your car, or office, meditating before returning home. An ideal solution would be for you both to meditate together at home, but that may not be possible.

To enhance the mood of contemplation and relaxation as you meditate, put a few drops of frankincense and myrrh in a vaporizer.

How to Meditate

First of all set the stage by finding a quiet place with as few distractions as possible. Once you are an expert you will be able to meditate in all sorts of different environments, but initially you need to be insulated from the outside world; no telephone, no doorbell, no one else in the room unless they are also meditating.

Sit in a comfortable place with a straight back, or kneel on a cushion. When the spine is straight your body is in balance and the least amount of effort is needed to sit upright. It is important there is no undue muscular tension. Don't lie down or you will probably fall asleep.

Close your eyes. Relax all your muscles, beginning with your feet and ending with your face. Breathe through your nose and become aware of your breathing. As you breathe out, repeat a phrase, word or sound, known as a mantra.*

Continue for 20 minutes. (It's okay to open your eyes to check the time.) When you finish sit quietly for several minutes, at first with your eyes closed, then with your eyes open.

Another technique which can be particularly effective is to sit and close your eyes as described above, and then concentrate on your breathing. Simply be totally aware of your abdomen slowly rising and falling with each breath. Gradually thoughts will fade away, and your mind will be at rest. You will be aware of everything going on around you, but will be peacefully detached.

---

* The purpose of repeating a word or a mantra is to divert your mind from extraneous thoughts. You can choose any word or sound. It is the repetition that helps keep your mind from wandering back to everyday problems. A soft meaningless sound is best—peace, seashore, one, aaahh, silence—but even your name can work. Tennyson is reputed to have meditated successfully by repeating his own name. Another method is to stare at a candle flame. It is, of course, the concentration on the word or flame that helps to empty your mind of disturbing thoughts.

The key to successful meditation is a passive attitude. You have to empty your mind of all thoughts and distractions. You need to sit quietly, still your mind and let your word float into your consciousness. And that, of course, for hyper, stressed-out people is very difficult. However, with practice it can be done. Don't worry if thoughts keep crowding in as you sit waiting for perfect peace. Gently bring your mind back to your special word, and gradually the thoughts will diminish. Even as they crowd in and you feel this is a waste of time, you are still reducing your stress level. All the stressful thoughts of the day are being gradually eliminated. Sometimes you may only attain a few minutes of total calm and peace; at others you may slip into inner calm immediately.

I had a very difficult time learning to meditate. Having read all the literature and the medical claims, I decided to try it. I took a series of lessons and ended up being thoroughly frustrated. I didn't feel any different after meditation, and inner calm during the 20-minute sessions eluded me. In fact, I found the whole thing pretty boring. However, people I respected, and who assured me it was great, persuaded me to continue. So, curbing my impatience, I persevered. After a couple of weeks, I began to get short periods of inner calm. However, the minute it happened, my conscious mind (which always seemed to be warily hovering) would kick in and say, "Wow, you made it." And the calm was gone.

The fact is, I finally made it. I can now meditate successfully, and it is excellent. It took me well over two months, but along the way I was gradually extending the periods of stillness. I found myself thinking of nothing, my muscles relaxed, and I experienced a sense of peaceful calm. So try not to be analytic as you meditate. Nothing is worse than your cynical self sitting to one side thinking how dumb this is. One of the problems for many people is all the mystical and spiritual overtones that have attached themselves to the practice. Visions of Eastern gurus in robes and beads and groups of flower children meditating may be off-putting. However, the claims of the gurus are supported by medical fact. Physiological changes take place in your body as you meditate. Stress and tension are dissipated. You will find yourself coping with stressful situations far more calmly.

Sex, Love and Relationships

❦

Nothing can relieve stress more than a loving relationship; whether it is with your spouse, partner, parents, siblings or a very close friend. To have someone who will sit down and listen sympathetically to your tales of the day's traumas can bring life back into perspective and cause a major drop in your stress level. Sex too can be perfect for relieving stress; the pleasures of the sexual act, and the wonderful feeling of release and peace afterwards can wipe out memories of the worst day at work.

However, unfortunately there is a dark side to all this. Relationships with your family and friends, as well as sex, can also do more to increase your stress level than even the worst day at work, or the most frustrating drive home. Children are a delight and relieve stress by diverting your mind, and making you laugh. However, a fretful baby that cries all night, a demanding toddler, or a difficult teenager can drive your frustration level up faster than almost any other thing. Because, of course, it's okay to curse your boss (under your breath if you want to keep your job), but you know it's not okay to feel the same way about one of your children. So the stress of the situation is compounded by your effort to suppress these feelings, and your extreme guilt at having felt them.

Similarly, an overtired brain, and an aching body can sometimes totally fail to respond to a partner's need, and cause tremendous stress upon the relationship. When you are having a difficult time at work, or facing domestic problems, things feel as if they are all going against you, and you are losing control. You begin to lose your self-esteem, and your sex hormone levels can fall, leading to a decrease in libido. At this point it becomes difficult to respond to the needs of your partner, and so your stress level increases. You feel inadequate. Not only are you under stress at work, now you can't even participate successfully in the sexual act.

On the other hand, when you feel loved, cared for, satisfied and secure, your self-esteem is high and your sex hormone levels are elevated. You feel good about life in general, and have greater physical energy and sex drive.

In the worst cases of extreme stress, women can experience increased premenstrual tension, vaginal dryness, and stress may even lead to infertility. While men may experience a decreased libido, impotence, and again this may lead to sterility. This is all the extreme, but even in its mildest form, stress can lead to a definite decline in sexual energy and enjoyment. It is difficult to keep your mind on the job at hand when your brain is still worrying about what happened in the last meeting you attended.

With both partners working, or one at home coping with some domestic difficulty, it can frequently happen that you are both tired, irritable and exhausted at the end of the day. In this situation, an unguarded, irritable remark may well provoke a reaction that compounds your stress level to an intolerable degree.

So what to do about it all? The answer isn't to become a hermit and avoid all human contact. If your only contact with the world is on the Internet, you are not ensuring a life safe from human stress. The answer is to understand your body and your feelings. Acknowledge the fact that after a tough day you need to relax, to really wind down. If you have a partner, you both need to think about this together and work out how you can relax on neutral ground before you get into heavy discussions, or make demands on each other.

Here are some of the things you can do to ensure that your relationships are a positive factor in your life. If you are having troubles with your partner, it is no good spending more time at work and avoiding the issue. You will only compound your stress level. Take a little time to work at the relationship. The rewards will be high. Nothing counteracts a stressful work situation more than a happy domestic life.

Oh, and by the way, if you don't think any of this is particularly important for relieving stress—well, not compared with fresh air, exercise and a good diet—think again. Resist the urge to skip the following paragraphs. They may well do wonders for you.

Improving Relationships

RECOGNIZE WHAT STRESS DOES TO YOU

One of the things you may not realize is that when you are under stress you can be a real pain in the butt to live with. You are short-tempered, irritable and impatient; whereas previously you had a sunny nature, were patient and understanding. The problem is that this has an effect on your partner who tends to reflect your irritability. So you consider your partner is being totally unreasonable. And just at the time when you most need patience and under-standing. Unfortunately, your whole attitude provokes hostility. Your partner may well be understanding for a while, but if it goes on over a long period, even the most patient person begins to act differently towards you.

So learn to recognize when you are under stress. You already know the signs: insomnia, tight neck and shoul-ders, upset stomach, headaches, etc. Make sure you don't add to your stress level by provoking your family and friends into getting mad with you, or you won't find solace among the people you would normally turn to for comfort.

IMPROVE COMMUNICATION

Communicating your feelings to other people isn't always easy, and it is even more difficult when you are dog-tired from an overload of work and lack of sleep. You probably assume that if you speak you can communicate. This isn't necessarily true, so it is better to start with the idea that it takes care and skill to communicate effectively within a relationship.

When you speak to your partner, you assume they understand what you mean and even understand your reason for saying it. Unfortunately, this is not always the case, and can lead to some stress-ridden situations. So check to make sure they understand, and by the same token don't assume you know what your partner is saying. Ask questions to make sure.

Good communication isn't only talking and listening. So when you are speaking to your partner, be aware of your tone of voice and body language. "Of course I agree with you," said in an icy tone with folded arms does not encourage your partner to continue the conversation, or to believe what you are saying.

AVOID BLAME

Avoid blaming your partner. Try using "I" statements rather than "you" statements. For example, "I was upset that you didn't get home in time for dinner," rather than, "You never phone to say you'll be late, and now dinner's ruined, and it's too late to go to the show." "I feel totally overloaded around the house. I don't know how I am going to be able to cope," rather than "Why don't you ever put the garbage out? Why do you loaf around while I do all the work?" Blaming your partner is inflammatory and leads to arguments. Try the gentle approach by expressing how you feel about something.

Choose a suitable time and place to air your concerns where you won't be interrupted. Don't do it when you are tired, when you've been drinking, or when you are in a crowd.

FIND THE TIME

I know you don't have any time, but somehow you need to make the time to communicate with your partner. Just a few minutes listening to each other when you first come home can make a tremendous difference to a relationship.

If the only time you talk is at bedtime after the children have gone to bed and you are exhausted, it is not a good time to bring up serious issues. It will probably lead to an argument and a sleepless night. Just what your stress level needs.

Consciously make the time to be together. Organize an evening out once a week. And don't tell me you can't afford a baby sitter. Remember, divorces are expensive. Spend a little money on your current relationship—he or she is well worth it. If you aren't interested in the movies, then go for a walk together—just the two of you, or go out to lunch, or to an art gallery. What was it you used to enjoy doing together that you haven't done for a long time because you are too busy? Then in a relaxed atmosphere you can talk about things that are important to you. Talk about your hopes and dreams for the future. Ask how your partner is doing at work, and really listen. Share your anxieties and concerns. Give each other positive feedback about the things that are great in life.

PAY COMPLIMENTS

Compliments make us feel good. So take the time to pay your partner a compliment. And learn to accept compliments gracefully—don't make your partner feel foolish for having paid you one. Simply say thanks and smile.

PREPARE FOR CHANGE

We all know that change is stressful. Obviously, unpleasant changes like losing your job or having an accident are stressful, but even pleasant changes like moving to a beautiful new home, getting married, or a promotion at work, can be stressful.

Although you know change will affect you, you may not be prepared for the extent of that effect. And more importantly, you don't generally appreciate the effect it has on your partner. You are so wrapped up in your new situation you spend little time noticing their reactions. Normally, traumatic changes will be shared initially—the death of a favorite child, or a favorite pet, will be something you can mourn together—but moving to a new neighborhood, the total disruption that a new baby brings, or the excitement of a major promotion may have differing degrees of effect on each of you. Take the time to notice how the change is affecting your partner. Discuss how you feel, and ask how they feel. And make sure you really listen to the answer.

Prepare for the change ahead of time. Obtain as much information as you can—knowing what is going to happen makes it far less traumatic.

If it has been an unpleasant, unexpected change, then start to plan for the future. Reassess what is important to you both. Ask yourself what you can and can't change. Then decide what you are going to achieve in the future. And put your plans into action.

Make sure that while the change is taking place—be it pleasant or unpleasant—you make time for relaxation to relieve the stress. Go for a walk, soak in a hot bath, listen to music.

AVOID CONFLICTS

When you are under stress, you will in all probability at some point get into an argument with your partner, or you will be desperately biting your tongue trying not to snap back when your exhausted partner comes home from work and lashes out at you with his or her tongue for no reason whatsoever.

If you recognize the remark or criticism is because your partner is totally stressed out, then make a conciliatory statement, and encourage them to relax for half an hour; don't lose your temper and tell them how unreasonable they are being. If they come home and treat you that way every day, that is a different matter. Find a nice quiet time when they are relaxed and tell them how much their behavior upsets you.

Inevitably, you will find times when your views conflict and you cannot agree. That's okay, you are two different people, and the differences are probably what attracted you to your partner in the first place. Agree to disagree on some points, and then seek neutral ground where you can agree. Just remember, it's not what you disagree about that causes the problem. It is how you handle the discussion about it that makes the difference.

BEWARE OF PERFECTIONISM

Wouldn't it be wonderful if everyone was as perfect as you and I? Or for that matter, wouldn't it be wonderful if we were perfect? Well, maybe, but the problem is constantly striving to be perfect—although a highly commendable goal—can also do horrible things to your health, stress level and relationships.

You've all been raised on a media diet of perfection. You are supposed to have perfect bodies, perfect teeth, and have to be perfectly exceptional in the business world.

You also believe that your relationships should be perfect. You have to be swept off your feet by the grand passion, be the perfect bride and groom, never grow tired of your partner and raise 2.4 perfect children. Which probably accounts for the huge divorce, or breakup, rate. It's downright exhausting just thinking about it, let alone trying to live that way.

Similarly, in the business world you are probably striving to be the world's greatest manager, engineer, analyst, salesman or whatever, and this puts a crushing burden on your body. In the good old days before the world gathered speed, you could take the time it needed to paint the Sistine Chapel. Striving for perfection was a realistic aim. Now it can frequently be unrealistic. You cannot be perfect at everything all the time, and also be highly productive. Something has to give. And all too frequently it's your personal life and your health that go by the wayside.

The stress you engender in yourself as you strive for perfection at work causes you to be irritable when you return home, and as your sleep and health in general suffer, you become more and more difficult to live with. So one or the other of you then decides it is time to move on and find the perfect partner. You know they exist—the media tells you so.

So why do we strive for perfection? Again, there is absolutely nothing wrong with wanting to achieve great things and be superior to your peers. We don't get too far in life if we are always ready to settle for second best.

However, if you are to keep your health and enjoy happy relationships, you must be realistic. You cannot be perfect at everything. World champion athletes may well have untidy bedrooms. It really doesn't matter.

The trick is to spread your resources. Focus on the most important things, and make sure they get 80% of your energy. Learn to live with a lesser degree of effort on things that really don't matter. If you are working flat out on a project at work, it isn't important if the lawn gets mowed only once every two weeks instead of once a week (or how about hiring a gardening service?). Don't try to be superman or superwoman. You may be achieving miracles in your own eyes, but maybe your partner, or your boss, is not so impressed.

Stressless Sex

When you are going through a tough time at work—the project is slipping, your boss is always on your case, the design doesn't work, the mail is burying you, the meetings seem to be wall-to-wall—you come home exhausted seeking peace, relaxation and relief. But when you get there you are greeted by a repeat performance of the day—the children are playing up, your partner is exhausted, dozens of chores hover over your head, and you still have to read that report before tomorrow's 8 A.M. meeting. Sound familiar? The same scenario exists for the home-bound partner—dealing with a young family all day, visiting a sick mother, fighting the traffic, etc. The first time you get to talk to each other without being interrupted by the family or the phone is at 11 P.M., and now one or other of you is demanding sex.

Sometimes it works wonders, but on others it degenerates into just another chore that must be completed.

Sex can, and should, be a wonderful shared experience that leaves you both feeling relaxed and energized. When sex is good it constantly reinforces and strengthens a relationship. The man feels more love, and the woman gets the love she may have been missing, while communication and intimacy increase. Needless to say, the stresses of the day dissolve and recede way into the background after a successful sexual experience.

WHY DOES SEX SOMETIMES INCREASE YOUR STRESS LEVEL?

Why then when sex is important in reducing stress, does it so often have the reverse effect, and lead to relationship problems, and an increase in your stress level?

The first thing to realize is that when you are under extreme stress your body may not be able to respond to your partner. This will cause consternation and dismay initially, and in all probability a rapidly deteriorating situation. Instead of approaching sex with pleasurable anticipa-

---

If you are experiencing problems with your sex life to the point where it is affecting your relationship, then I urge you to contact a professional relationship counselor, therapist or medical practitioner. Talking the problem over with an objective and sympathetic third party can solve even severe problems.

tion, you will be worrying about your performance, and your stress level may rise to the point where your body cannot respond. A whole industry of sex therapists and counselors has grown helping people deal with serious problems that start from a simple overload of stress at work or in the home.

To enjoy sex you must be relaxed. Using sex as a release mechanism may work short term, but frequently ends up damaging a relationship. I realize when you are being constantly subjected to stress, it is impractical to assume you will be in a totally relaxed state when you go to bed at night. However, if you are going flat out all day, and through the evening, and the only time you have for sex is at 11 P.M. when you are both totally exhausted, you are probably not enjoying a wonderful sex life. Do you find the only time that sex is really great is when you are on vacation, when you are both relaxed and have time for each other? There is a clue in there somewhere. Try a little relaxation every day and things will improve dramatically.

To relieve stress, sex needs to be an enjoyable event for both parties. You should be able to relax and have a good time. If you are uptight and worrying about what might go wrong, you are on a downward spiral. So here are a few tips.

LIGHTEN UP

First of all, don't get too intense about sex. It doesn't have to be a monumental event each time. Orchestras don't have to play and the earth move. It should though be a pleasant shared experience. So keep your sense of humor and a lighthearted approach. It is supposed to be fun, after all.

If your partner is going through a particularly stressful period at work, be sympathetic. Perhaps all you need to do is lie down and talk to each other and cuddle. Give each other warmth and support. Sex may or may not follow. It isn't too important at this stage. When your partner knows they can relax with you, and are not forced to perform, paradoxically they again become capable of performing.

STRIKE A BALANCE

An overtired man wants sex to release the frustrations of the day. He is quickly aroused, and can indulge in sex and be sound asleep in half an hour. Terrific. Not so terrific for his partner, however. She may be completely turned off, and end up downright frustrated. So reach a compromise. First of all, talk about it. Not during the sexual encounter, but at some time when you are both in a relaxed state of mind. Then take whatever steps you need to get into the mood. Sounds nasty and clinical, doesn't it? It isn't. It's important to your relationship, and it has surprisingly pleasant results. The problem is that most couples only discuss sex when things are going wrong, and then it turns into a very heavy discussion. So talk about it as soon as possible. Keep the conversation light and friendly (it's okay to laugh about it too), but bring small concerns out into the open before they turn into something major. Make sure if you voice a concern you do it in a very positive way. The male of the species is particularly and acutely sensitive to criticism where sex is concerned. So make sure you couch things in the terms of "I really like that" versus "I hate that."

FIND THE TIME FOR SEX

When you are flat out at work and every evening is full, sex tends to take place at the end of the day when you go to bed, or on Sunday mornings. And often it becomes less and less frequent. Of course, you are now responsible, grown- up people with a million domestic responsibilities, frequent sex is for new partners and adolescents.

Have you noticed you have time to watch TV every evening, or pursue mindless conversations on the Internet? You find time to go to the gym or the swimming pool. You have time to talk to your friends on the phone, go to a movie, go out to dinner, but you don't have time for sex.

I have news for you. You do have time for sex, and it can be very enjoyable. All you need to do is work it into your schedule. Switch off the TV news—the world will get along without you—send the kids over to mother's for the evening, or hire a sitter to take them all out to the movies, then open up a bottle of wine and relax together.

If the only time that sex is enjoyable is when you are on vacation, then set up a mini-vacation on a regular basis. Go away for the weekend. A new environment, free of all the chores and anxieties of home can work wonders. You will also find that on the long drive to your destination, you have time to talk. And communication is an essential part of a happy relationship.

Or if you have young children and never have any time together, hire a babysitter and go out to a hotel for the evening. Outrageous? Yes, but probably not much more expensive than dinner and a movie.

TRY A LITTLE ROMANCE

The old truism that men hunger for sex and women for romance is surprisingly true. Even in this day and age of power-hungry, goal-oriented professional women, women still like some romance in their lives. There's a billion dollar romance novel industry out there to prove it. Unfortunately, a lot of men don't realize this or at least can't understand it. They know when they are getting to know a woman that chocolates, candlelit dinners and romantic locations work, but it all seems so unnecessary when they're going to go to bed with her regularly. If your relationship has reached the dull, flat, stale and ordinary stage, try bringing a little romance into it. It will work wonders.

AFFAIRS AREN'T THE ANSWER

While on the subject of relationships becoming dull, flat and ordinary, let's talk about affairs. They're exciting, stimulating and fun. All the thrill of illicit sex and a new partner. However, they can also add dramatically to your stress level both during the affair and in its aftermath.

It is strange how stressed-out people who don't have time to make their current relationships work can find the time to chase another person, and arrange meeting places. Investing the same time and energy in turning your current relationship into something exciting pays far higher dividends. Start having some fun in your life within your current relationship. Stop taking it so seriously.

If it's the illicit bit that turns you on, then lock your bedroom door and indulge in sex while the children or your parents are in the living room. Check into a motel for the night under an assumed name. Use your imagination.

KEEPING FIT PAYS OFF

You need to be reasonably fit to enjoy sex. If all you do is eat, smoke and watch TV after work, you may find your interest in sex diminishing. This is not the effect of being in a dull relationship, or of advancing years, it's sheer physical inertia. So get out for that 15-minute walk in the evening, start eating properly and cut back (or preferably cut out) smoking, and have fun with sex instead.

AVOID OLYMPIC SEX

Unfortunately in our current goal-oriented society where success is all important, and being the absolute best at everything is paramount, even sex does not escape. People read books on sexual techniques, watch porno movies where the participants achieve incredible feats, and listen to the exploits of the neighborhood stud in the locker room at the gym. It's enough to give anyone an inferiority complex. Or worse yet, they are so focused on their technique, they totally lose sight of the fact it's supposed to be an enjoyable experience. It really doesn't matter how often you have sex, or how long you indulge in it, no one is keeping a scorecard. Only you. Relax, leave the competitive stresses behind, and have a good time.

A Few More Ideas

I n this chapter I touch on a few more things for you to think about. Nothing that requires any action on your part. The exception is the first item—biofeedback. I've given a brief overview and suggest you talk to your doctor if you would like to try it.

Biofeedback

If you would like some scientific help in learning how to relax, then you might try biofeedback. Relaxing is associated with several physiological changes in the body. The heart rate and breath rate are decreased, and blood pressure falls. The whole of the sympathetic nervous system is dampened down, causing muscles to relax and use less oxygen. And another non-obvious change is that the amount of sweat produced by our skin is significantly reduced.

Sweat reduction is used in most biofeedback techniques. Although small changes in sweat production cannot easily be measured, this change brings about a secondary change in the skin's resistance to the passage of an electric current. These electrical changes are turned into an audio signal by means of an electrical device built into a biofeedback monitoring unit.

During biofeedback sessions you are asked to lie on a couch dressed in comfortable clothing and go through a series of relaxation routines such as controlled breathing, muscle relaxation routines or some form of meditation. Two finger electrodes are fitted which connect to the biofeedback monitoring unit. The unit is tuned so that a steady sound signal is broadcast. As the relaxation procedures begin to take effect, the note of the transmitter either changes or stops altogether. Biofeedback sessions are generally for half an hour a week over a period of three months.

Blood pressure can be brought down substantially by biofeedback, and even the severity of migraine attacks can be mitigated. Obviously it can also be used to monitor how successfully you are mastering the relaxation techniques. It is a serious scientific approach to the whole problem of learning to relax, but unquestionably you can achieve the same results without an electronic aid. However, if you are interested, I suggest you talk to your family doctor who will be able to give you the names of clinics and hospitals where it is carried out.

In the meantime, do be patient with yourself as you learn to relax. Unconsciously you have become tense and uptight as a result of stress. However, unless you now find yourself in a stress-free situation, you are going to consciously have to learn to relax. It has taken a while to reach your present state, so by the same token it will take a while for the relaxation techniques to take effect. Always bear in mind that, although you may not instantly feel relaxed and euphoric, the techniques described will be working to undo the harmful effects of stress. So don't be hard on yourself if you don't achieve instantaneous results. It will take a little time. Be patient, keep at it; you are on your way to feeling great.

Humor

Remember the old wives' tale "Laughter is the best medicine." It is. Nothing relaxes stress more than laughter. Think how good you feel after you have spent time with someone who makes you laugh a lot.

So go and see funny movies, watch sitcoms that appeal to your sense of humor or read humorous books. And, if you have a friend or partner who makes you laugh, cherish them and make sure you spend time with them.

In World War II everyone marveled at the Cockneys in inner London who survived the traumas and stresses of night after night of bombing. They seldom got a complete night's sleep because they had to leave their homes and hurry to underground shelters. They sat there as the planes dropped their bombs and the artillery pounded away. Next morning they emerged, not sure what they would find. Their house gone? Their neighbors killed? Yet they all went to work every day and few of them cracked under the strain. If ever you have been around Cockneys you would know why. They have a great sense of humor and laugh about everything. And the worse things get, the more they find to laugh about.

Remember, it takes less muscular
energy to smile than to frown

Appearance

We frequently create stress for ourselves totally unnecessarily. And all too often because of how we think we look. We feel too fat or too thin, or our hair needs doing. We are convinced other people are looking at us critically and noticing that our nose is too long or our eyes are too close set.

In fact, people don't see these details. They react to you, the whole person. Your bearing, your presence, your confidence and your personality. So stop worrying about things you can do nothing about. Instead, stand tall, be proud of yourself. Wear bright, positive colors if you feel mousy. Or soft pastels if you feel too aggressive.

Lighten Up

Life really isn't that serious. Try regarding it as something to enjoy. Greg Norman is the world's highest paid golfer, and yet he has never won the Masters—one of golf's most prestigious tournaments. Somehow it always eludes him. In 1996, he went into the last round six strokes up on Nick Faldo, his closest competitor. At last he was going to win the title. Yet by the end of the day he had totally blown it and was once again the runner up. The press mobbed him, asking him how he felt, sure he must be devastated. He simply looked them in the eye, and said, "Well, the sun's going to come up tomorrow again."

At one stage in my career, I had the world's worst boss. He was a regular pain in the butt, and I used to go home at night tearing my hair out in frustration at his latest stupid decision. I couldn't imagine how I was going to survive. I considered giving up a job I loved in order to get away from him. Then one day it suddenly struck me. I only had to put up with him at work. Each night I went home to a charming husband, while my boss went home to his wife. From there on in, whenever he gave me a bad time, I would grin inwardly. Imagine having to live with him. I started to enjoy my job again, and eventually he moved on.

Fishing

One of my favorite activities is fishing. It was one of the ways a hyper type like me could relax (before I discovered all the neat things we've been talking about). When you're fishing, you can stand staring vacantly at the sea or river, and no one makes you feel guilty (least of all yourself) about doing nothing. After all, a fish might bite. You never know when it is going to happen, so you're in a state of calm, relaxed alertness. Now isn't that what meditation is all about?

Right After Work

Most people feel the greatest amount of stress at the end of the working day. All the problems of the day accumulate, leaving tense, aching shoulders, pounding head, etc., and now you have to rush home and get dinner, pick up the kids or whatever. Small wonder your stress count goes up.

So as you commute home, put on relaxing music (by pressing a pre-tuned switch), do breathing exercises at traffic lights and, as you travel, breathe in the aroma of the lavender oil you wiped across the dashboard before going to work in the morning. The sun has heated the oil and the car smells wonderful.

When you arrive home, do you really need to start dinner right away, or the laundry, or make phone calls. Take twenty minutes to yourself and go for a walk in the park, slip into a warm scented bath, or meditate. Your whole evening will take on a different complexion. And your partner, children and pets are going to like the relaxed you. Even the pile of work you brought home will go more smoothly.

Emile Coué

If your mind is beginning to boggle at all the things you can do to relieve stress, you may either turn to the next chapter which outlines a few standard approaches you can do by rote, or you can think a little about good old Emile Coué. Emile was a French pharmacist, born in Troyes in 1857. He found fame and fortune in the 1920s when he set up a clinic in Nancy based on the realization of the powers of auto-suggestion. His lectures in England and the U.S. attracted a great deal of attention and his followers were reputed to be in the millions. He maintained that the unconscious self dictates all our functions and that auto-suggestion could cure almost anything that ailed us.

Perhaps his popularity, and his true claim to fame, was the simplicity of his system. Every morning on waking, and every night before sleeping, he said you should shut your eyes and repeat 20 times—while moving the lips and mechanically counting knots on a string—the words, "Every day in every respect I am getting better and better." The key was the degree of concentration and the confidence and faith with which this mantra was repeated.

Coué believed his system worked by wiping out the conscious mind, while the subconscious stayed awake and receptive and could be spoken to. So if all else fails, buy a piece of string and remember Emile.

Compartmentalize Your Life

We've talked about Chinese philosophy and the necessity for balance in your life. To learn to cope with stress, you must adjust your lifestyle. You need exercise, good nutrition and you need to practice some of the techniques that have been described.

To deal with stress, you must take time for yourself. Find balance. Compartmentalize your life so that you have time for work, time for your family, time to sleep and time in which you can relax. It is going to take a little time to organize it, but it is essential. Life is to be enjoyed, and with balance it can be.

I am well aware how difficult it is when both you and your partner are flat out at work all week and you have a mountain of chores on the weekend. Even when you get home at night and would love to sit with your feet up, you have to run around and start preparing a meal, or check your kids' homework or whatever. If you are living alone, it can be even more difficult. But there are solutions. None of you would be in the positions you are today if you weren't smart. I bet your last evaluation even mentioned how well organized you are. Okay, so now is the time to use those smarts to improve your own lifestyle. Start thinking innovatively. Are there things you are doing you could get someone else to do? Just because your father always fixed his own car and changed the washers in the tap doesn't mean you have to. If your mother baked cakes, mowed the lawn and replaced tiles on the roof after a storm, it doesn't mean you need to do the same. Think about a little delegation. There are people whose livelihood depends on someone employing them to do these things. Start to spread the wealth around!

For years I worked ridiculous hours at work, brought work home with me in the evenings and, in addition, cooked meals each night, cleaned the house, and did the garden on the weekend. Of course, my husband and son helped, but I always felt the home was my responsibility and if the house was a mess (which it was most of the time) it was my fault. I started to think how wonderful it would be to have a housekeeper, but we couldn't really afford one and I wasn't sure I wanted someone around the house all the time.

Then some genius suggested I advertise for part-time help. It was unbelievable. I got dozens of replies. There are a lot of people out there who need extra money but who can't cope with a full-time job. So I ended up with a marvelous woman, a grandmother, who arrived at ten each day and left at two. She picked up groceries, cooked dinner and cleaned the house. We all came home to a clean house and dinner sitting waiting to be heated up. It was fantastic. My husband and son started to quite like me now that I wasn't constantly grumbling at them to get chores done on the weekend. I started to get more fresh air and exercise and began to feel really good about life. Needless to say, I was far more effective at work. Promotions and money followed and the housekeeper's salary was more than covered.

Your circumstances will all be different. But there is one thing you must do, and that is apply your mind to solving the problems that lie between you and an enjoyable, healthy lifestyle. Simply decide you are going to do it and then solve the problems. Once you have made up your mind and have the objective firmly in mind, you will get there.

Finding the Time

You'll be reading all these ideas for building up your immunity to stress and thinking they sound good, but I don't have any time now. That's half the problem. How am I going to find time to linger in warm baths, walk in the sunshine and sit still for twenty minutes meditation?

The fact is to achieve a well-balanced lifestyle takes effort. However, it is mainly a question of reorganizing your life to fit in the things that are important. So take a day off this weekend or, if that is too crowded already, then take a vacation day and spend the time thinking through ways of finding the time.

You will find, for example, that if you get up 30 minutes earlier each day and exercise, you will improve the quality of your sleep and feel more refreshed and rested even with 30 minutes less time in bed.

ELEVEN

Summary

In this chapter, I will summarize a few of the main points you need to consider if you are going to get stress under control, and then give a step-by-step approach to get you started. Although, as I mentioned earlier, you can use any of the techniques that appeal to you, in any order. There is no set approach that will necessarily work for everyone. However, I would suggest you start to get some exercise—a short walk will be fine—and make sure you are eating properly (plenty of fresh fruit and vegetables) because without a healthy body all the other techniques are far less effective.

The important thing is to enjoy getting stress under control. Most of the techniques suggested are fun to try. So mix and match, and come up with your own stress reduction cocktail.

Basic Facts About Stress

1. The level of stress you experience is directly related to your reaction to stress. You can lessen the effects of stress by learning to modify your reactions. When you react less, the physical problems generated by stress are substantially reduced.

2. Physiological changes in the body occur when you are in a stressful situation. The "fight or flight" response causes changes in the body's chemistry, increasing alertness, muscular strength and speed to prepare for a physical showdown, or a hasty retreat. When you are subjected to long-term, psychological stress, your body still initiates the fight or flight response, but with no physical release, your body stays on red alert for extended periods, and you are unable to relax.

It is possible to counteract the effects of stress by initiating the relaxation response. The fight or flight response programs your body for action, the relaxation response deprograms it, dissipating the effects of stress before it can harm you. The relaxation response is based on the principle that when you are anxious or disturbed your muscles tense. When muscles relax, the mind relaxes, and the tension caused by stress quickly fades away.

The relaxation response is initiated by:
• Controlled breathing.
• Meditation.
• Aromatherapy—soothing essential oils absorbed by the body—through the nose by inhalation, or through the skin by massage.

- Reflexology—massaging the reflex points in the foot.
- Exercise.

3. To help your body in the fight against stress you need to pay attention to your diet, and ensure that you are getting the correct nutrients. A brain starved of nutrients is ill equipped to deal with mental stress.

4. Treating the symptoms of stress is not the answer. You need to get down to the basic causes. Take responsibility for your own body and your own life. Learn to control your reaction to stress, and to nullify its effects by initiating the relaxation response, but also treat your body right with good food and refreshing exercise. Then take a long, hard look at your lifestyle. Are you spending enough time on the things, and with the people, you enjoy? Squander a whole day and consider how you can cut out some of the things that cause you stress, and make time for the things you enjoy. It may be as simple as getting household help, a garden service, going to the car wash instead of doing it yourself, or learning how to relax at the airport when the plane is late.

5. One of the most severe symptoms of stress is chronic fatigue, mainly caused by lack of, or disturbed, sleep. Go to bed at a regular time each night, even on the weekends. Program your body to be tired at a certain time each night. You already have it programmed for mealtimes. Relax for brief periods during the day so that you are not always tense at bedtime. Read the tips on sleep in Chapter 4, and practice some of them. They don't take up much time, and they will pay dividends. And remember, lack of sleep does you no harm (other than make you feel tired), tossing and turning and fretting over lack of sleep does harm you. So relax, and sleep will come.

Step-by-Step Techniques

1. Take a brisk 20-minute walk before work, or at lunchtime, or any other form of exercise you enjoy. Exercise will release the tension in your muscles.

2. Practice controlled breathing at traffic lights, at home, or in the office. Breathe in on the count of seven, and then exhale slowly on the count of 15. As you breathe in, push out your abdomen and feel the oxygen expanding your chest, then slowly exhale, feeling the tension drain out of you. Repeat five or more times. Don't worry if you can't make it to 15 to start with. Eight will do for starters. Taking a very deep breath after a disturbing phone call, or lethal meeting, will bring down your stress level.

3. Pre-program your car radio to a station that plays classical or soothing music. Or stock up on relaxing tapes. Let the music soothe you as you drive to and from work.

4. Start eating more fresh fruit and vegetables. Cut down on fatty foods, highly processed foods containing white flour and white sugar, caffeine and excessive alcohol. Your body is going into basic training to tackle the stress monster.

5. Pick up some essential oils from the health food store next time you are out shopping: a carrier, or base oil, of sweet almond or saffola, and lavender, bergamot, cedarwood, sandalwood, or any pre-mixed relaxation oils recommended by the health food store. Make sure the oils you buy are pure, essential oils. Chapter 5 lists several oils that help you relax if you don't feel energetic enough to select your own.

Take a warm, relaxing bath either when you first get home or before bed, and feel the warmth of the water combined with the benefits of the essential oils melt away muscle tension and relax the mind. Make sure the water is warm (97-101 degrees F.), not hot, and windows are closed to get the maximum benefit from the oils. Put a handful of bath salts into the tub and add 3 drops of lavender, 3 drops of bergamot and 2 drops of cedarwood, swish them around, then get in and enjoy for 15 minutes.

6. Wipe some lavender oil on the dashboard of your car in the morning so it is filled with the soothing aroma of lavender when you drive home in the evening.

7. Improve the quality of your sleep by cutting down on caffeine and colas, and listening to soothing music just before you go to sleep. Don't watch violent videos or disturbing TV in the evening, and try to avoid arguments at bedtime. If you can't get to sleep after twenty minutes, or you wake up in the night and can't get back to sleep, don't toss and turn. Get up and read for a while. Have a glass of milk. Let your body cool down. When you go back to your warm, comfortable bed, you'll drop right off.

8. Talk your partner, or a friend, into giving you a neck and shoulder massage using 12 ml of sweet almond oil as the carrier oil, and 5 drops of lavender essential oil, and 1 drop sandalwood. Pour the sweet almond oil into a glass container—never use plastic containers for essential oils— add the essential oils and mix. Apply a thin layer so that the skin glows but is not greasy. Continue to massage until the oil is absorbed. If you live on your own or your partner's away, you can always give yourself a foot massage. That makes you feel great.

These few items are just to get you started. I would encourage you to skip back through the book and try a few more things. Really work on your sleep patterns (Chapter 4) because once you are sleeping well, and waking refreshed every morning, you are going to be able to find more time for yourself.

How to Give a Massage

❧❦❧

The art of massage can be learned from the many books on the subject or, if you haven't got time to pick up a book on massage, here are the basic essentials. Massage therapists use a special table, but a futon or padded floor will work at home. Beds are not firm enough. A large bath or beach towel covered with a cotton sheet works well for both futon and floor. Another towel will be needed to cover up the person being massaged. Make sure the room is sufficiently heated, light is diffused and outside noise is at a minimum. Soft background music can enhance a feeling of relaxation.

The person giving the massage should remove jewelry or watches that might scratch and it is important that he or she is relaxed. Tense fingers have a tendency to dig into flesh and cause discomfort.

Giving a massage can be as relaxing for the person giving the massage as for the recipient. Provided you start out in a calm state of mind and become totally absorbed in the massage strokes, you will find yourself growing increasingly relaxed, which will in turn transmit itself to your partner.

Sweet almond oil or coconut oil can be used for the base oil blended with your favorite essential oil. Warm oil and hands before massage. Keep oil in a bowl and dip fingers in it rather than pouring from a jug. Massage strokes should be slow and gentle, each movement blending into the next. Always towards the heart, from extremities to body center. This encourages the flow of blood to the heart.

Maintain constant contact during massage.

Keep extremities and areas not being worked on warm.

Avoid applying pressure directly to the spine and joints.

The person being massaged should eat lightly before massage and drink plenty of water afterwards.

If a full body massage is going to take too long, or is too exhausting for the person giving the massage, practice back massages. They're easy to do and don't take long. And they feel good. Pay special attention to the neck area and lower back where tension and stress are stored.

One of the major benefits of using natural products for massage is that the body has a great affinity with natural

---

Essential oils in the pure state are too highly concentrated to be used directly on the skin. They should be diluted in a base or carrier oil.

PREPARING AN
ANTI-STRESS MASSAGE OIL

2 tablespoons sweet almond or coconut oil

10 drops lavender essential oil

2 drops neroli or rose essential oil

Pour sweet almond or coconut oil into a glass or glazed ceramic bowl (never use plastic containers for essential oils). Add essential oils. This amount of massage oil will provide a fine layer so that the skin glows but is not greasy. Continue to massage until the oil is absorbed. Leave the oil on your body after massage for further absorption and benefit from the tranquilizing effects of the essential oils. If you give yourself a mini-massage in the morning, wear a toweling robe afterwards while you get ready for work and eat breakfast. This will give the oil a few more minutes to be absorbed before you get dressed.

ingredients, and the oils can enter and leave the body, leaving no toxins behind.

Foot Massage

You can either massage your own feet or have someone massage them for you. Remove your shoes and socks or tights, and sit comfortably. If you are massaging your own feet, make sure you are not straining your back as you work on your feet. If you are supple enough to bend one knee and put your foot on your lap, that's great. If not, don't worry. Use one of the massage oils recommended under Aromatherapy, Chapter 5, or almond oil or any lotion that will let your hands slip easily over your feet will work. Of course, if you use an aromatherapy blend, you are doubling up the relaxation benefits.

You need to use both hands to massage effectively. One hand massages while the other hand supports the foot. Put four fingers on the top of the foot and the thumb on the sole (reverse finger and thumb position for self-massage); the supporting hand should always stay close to the working hand. Always keep the foot bent slightly towards you in a comfortable grip—not too tightly or with the toes bent backwards.

Now press firmly on a pressure point with your thumb and rotate it two or three times. The thumb should be bent from the joint at a 75 to 90 degree angle; the nail should not press into the flesh. The contact point is the tip of the thumb. After rotating the thumb, lift it and move. The movement should be small, so that you are working progressively, covering every inch of the foot. The basic procedure is: press in, rotate two or three times, lift and move. It is a good idea to practice the rotating movement on your hand before getting started on your first foot.

To relieve stress, start by massaging the reflex area on the foot that corresponds to the solar plexus. A great deal of tension is stored in the solar plexus. Once the solar plexus is relaxed, you can breathe more deeply, allowing the bottom of the lungs to expand which releases tension at a deep level. This makes response to further treatment more effective. To locate the solar plexus reflex, grasp the top of the foot at the metatarsal area and squeeze gently. A

REFLEXOLOGY

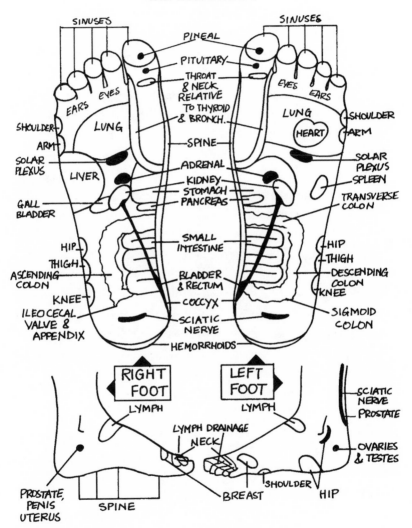

depression will appear on the sole of the foot at the midpoint of the base of the ball of the foot. This is the solar plexus reflex. Inhale as you press in on this point, and exhale as you release pressure. Repeat several times.

Next, cup the back of the ankle of the right foot in the palm of the left hand, with the thumb on the outside of the ankle and the fingers on the inside (reverse finger and thumb position for self-massage). With your other hand, grasp the foot at the base of the big toe (thumb on sole of foot and fingers on top) and rotate gently, first in one direction, and then in the other. Maneuver the foot as far as it will go comfortably. The foot should be as relaxed and passive as possible with the hands doing all the work. The objective is to loosen any stiffness in the ankle. Don't force the ankle.

The toes represent the head and neck area. By rotating them you will release tension and loosen muscles in the neck and shoulders. The principle is the same as ankle rotation.

Support the foot with one hand as you rotate each toe in turn. The supporting hand should firmly hold the base of each toe as it is rotated. With the massage hand, hold the toe close to the base joint with the thumb below and index and third finger on top. Rotate each toe clockwise and anti-clockwise a few times.

With one hand, hold the top of your foot to steady it, and make a fist with the other hand. Place your fist on the ball of your foot and stroke all the way down the sole of your foot. Return your fist to the ball of the foot and repeat at least six times. This is very relaxing since it is equivalent to massaging the whole body.

These massaging techniques will help relieve tension, but they are not a substitute for the work of a reflexologist. To obtain the maximum benefit, it is better to invest an hour with a professional (if of course you have an hour!).

Index